JOYDEEP ROY

USMLE Step 3 Review

1st Edition

GW00708672

USMLE Step 3 Review

1st Edition

225

Questions & Answers

Carlyle H. Chan, MD, FAPA
Associate Professor
Director of Residency Education and
Continuing Medical Education
Department of Psychiatry and Behavioral Medicine
Medical College of Wisconsin
Milwaukee, Wisconsin

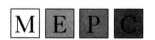

APPLETON & LANGE
Stamford, Connecticut

Notice: The authors and the publisher of this volume have taken care to make certain that the doses of drugs and schedules of treatment are correct and compatible with the standards generally accepted at the time of publication. Nevertheless, as new information becomes available, changes in treatment and in the use of drugs become necessary. The reader is advised to carefully consult the instruction and information material included in the package insert of each drug or therapeutic agent before administration. This advice is especially important when using new or infrequently used drugs. The authors and publisher disclaim all responsibility for any liability, loss, injury, or damage incurred as a consequence, directly or indirectly, of the use and application of any of the contents of the volume.

Copyright © 1997 by Appleton & Lange
A Simon & Schuster Company

All rights reserved. This book, or any parts thereof, may not be used or reproduced in any manner without written permission. For information, address Appleton & Lange, Four Stamford Plaza, PO Box 120041, Stamford, Connecticut 06912-0041.

97 98 99 00 01 / 10 9 8 7 6 5 4 3 2 1

Prentice Hall International (UK) Limited, *London*
Prentice Hall of Australia Pty. Limited, *Sydney*
Prentice Hall Canada, Inc., *Toronto*
Prentice Hall Hispanoamericana, S.A., *Mexico*
Prentice Hall of India Private Limited, *New Delhi*
Prentice Hall of Japan, Inc., *Tokyo*
Simon & Schuster Asia Pte. Ltd., *Singapore*
Editora Prentice Hall do Brasil Ltda., *Rio de Janeiro*
Prentice Hall, *Upper Saddle River, New Jersey*

ISBN 0-8385-6339-2

ISBN: 0-8385-6339-2
ISSN: 1090-3631

9 780838 563397   90000

Acquisitions Editor: Marinita Timban
Production Editor: Lisa M. Guidone
Production Service: Inkwell Publishing Services
Designer: Libby Schmitz

PRINTED IN THE UNITED STATES OF AMERICA

APPLETON & LANGE
QUICK REVIEW SERIES

Health Related

MEPC: Medical Assistant
Examination Review, 5/e
Durham
1996, ISBN 0-8385-6230-2

MEPC: Medical Record,
Examination Review, 6/e
Bailey
1994, ISBN 0-8385-6192-6

**MEPC: Occupational
Therapy**
Examination Review, 5/e
Dundon
1988, ISBN 0-8385-7204-9

MEPC: Optometry
Examination Review, 4/e
Casser et al.
1994, ISBN 0-8385-7449-1

**MEPC: Physician
Assistant**
Examination Review, 3/e
Rahr and Niebuhr
1996, ISBN 0-8385-8094-7

Comprehensive
A & L Reviews

**MEPC: USMLE Step 1
Review**
Fayemi
1995, ISBN 0-8385-6269-8

**MEPC: USMLE Step 2
Review**
Jacobs
1996, ISBN 0-8385-6270-1,
A6270-1

**MEPC: USMLE Step 3
Review**
Chan
1996, ISBN 0-8385-6339-2,
A6339-4

Basic Science

MEPC: Anatomy, 10/e
A USMLE STEP 1 Review
Wilson
1995, ISBN 0-8385-6218-3

MEPC: Biochemistry, 11/e
A USMLE STEP 1 Review
Glick
1995, ISBN 0-8385-5779-1

MEPC: Microbiology, 11/e
A USMLE Step 1 Review
Kim
1995, ISBN 0-8385-6308-2

MEPC: Pathology, 10/e
A USMLE STEP 1 Review
Fayemi
1994, ISBN 0-8385-8441-1

MEPC: Pharmacology, 8/e
A USMLE STEP 1 Review
Krzanowski et al.
1995, ISBN 0-8385-6227-2

MEPC: Physiology, 9/e
A USMLE STEP 1 Review
Penney
1995, ISBN 0-8385-6222-1

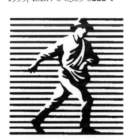

Clinical Science

MEPC: Neurology, 10/e
A USMLE Step 2 Review
Slosberg
1993, ISBN 0-8385-5778-3

MEPC: Pediatrics, 9/e
A USMLE Step 2 Review
Hansbarger
1995, ISBN 0-8385-6223-X

**MEPC: Preventive
Medicine and Public
Health, 10/e**
A USMLE Step 2 Review
Hart
June 1996, ISBN 0-8385-
6319-8

MEPC: Psychiatry, 10/e
A USMLE Step 2 Review
Chan and Prosen
1995, ISBN 0-8385-5780-5

MEPC: Surgery, 11/e
A USMLE Step 2 Review
Metzler
1995, ISBN 0-8385-6195-0

Specialty Board
Reviews

**MEPC: Anesthesiology,
9/e**
Specialty Board Review
Dekornfeld and Sanford
1995, ISBN 0-8385-0256-3

MEPC: Otolaryngology
Specialty Board Review
Head & Neck Surgery
Willett and Lee
1995, ISBN 0-8385-7580-3

MEPC: Neurology, 4/e
Specialty Board Review
Giesser and Kanof
1995, ISBN 0-8385-8650-3

To order or for more information, visit your local health science bookstore

or call Appleton & Lange toll free

1-800-423-1359

CONTENTS

CONTRIBUTING EDITORS

Carlyle H. Chan, MD, FAPA
Associate Professor
Director of Residency Education and
    Continuing Medical Education
Department of Psychiatry and Behavioral Medicine
Medical College of Wisconsin
Milwaukee, Wisconsin

Geoffrey Lamb, MD
Associate Professor
Department of General Internal Medicine
Medical College of Wisconsin
Director, Ambulatory Care Clinic
Froedert Hospital
Milwaukee, Wisconsin

Loren Leshan, MD
Associate Professor
Department of Family and Community Medicine
Medical College of Wisconsin
Residency Director
St. Mary's Hospital Family Medicine Program
Milwaukee, Wisconsin

Len Scarpinato, DO, FAAFP
Associate Professor
Department of Family and Community Medicine
Medical College of Wisconsin
Critical Care Curriculum Coordinator
St. Mary's Hospital Family Medicine Program
Milwaukee, Wisconsin

Gary Swart, MD, FACEP
Assistant Professor and Residency Director
Department of Emergency Medicine
Medical College of Wisconsin
Milwaukee, Wisconsin

Karen Wendelberger, MD
Associate Professor and Vice Chair of Education
Director of the Critical Care Fellowship Program
Department of Pediatrics
Medical College of Wisconsin
Vice Chief of Staff
Children's Hospital of Wisconsin
Milwaukee, Wisconsin

PREFACE

Step 3 of the United States Medical Licensing Examination (USMLE) is the final test of medical knowledge and clinical science understanding before licensure. The newly revised examination has been organized around clinical encounter frames and physician tasks.

This review book has followed the instructions and content description in the Bulletin for the USMLE Step 3. The concise answers have the most recent references as source material. All questions are of the best answer format with some multiple item sets of two to three consecutive questions based on the same clinical material or clinical clusters of four to nine consecutive questions. The questions have been grouped into five clinical settings: office, hospital, emergency department, satellite health center, and other encounters that span a large cross-section of knowledge and tasks.

We believe this review will assist you in your preparation for this important exam and will aid in assessing your strengths and weaknesses. We hope you agree.

I would like to acknowledge Appleton & Lange's editorial staff of Marinita Timban and Amy Schermerhorn for their assistance. I would also like to recognize my administrative assistants, Dasha Haas and Kelli Prince, for their help. Finally, I would like to extend my appreciation to my wife, Patricia, and my children, Christopher and Diana, for their sacrifice of several weekends during the preparation of this book.

Carlyle H. Chan, MD, FAPA

1

Office

DIRECTIONS (Questions 1–69): Each of the numbered items or incomplete statements in this chapter is followed by answers or completions of the statement. Select the **ONE** lettered answer or completion that is **BEST** in each case.

Case Cluster (Questions 1–3):
Refer to Figure 1.1.

1. A 28-year-old woman presents to the office with complaints of fatigue. She has been chewing ice and her grandmother told her she might have "low blood." Family history is significant for anemia. What would **NOT** be consistent with the peripheral blood smear in Figure 1.1?

    A. Sideroblastic anemias

    B. Thalassemia

    C. Iron deficiency

    D. Sickle cell disease

    E. Autoimmune hemolytic anemia

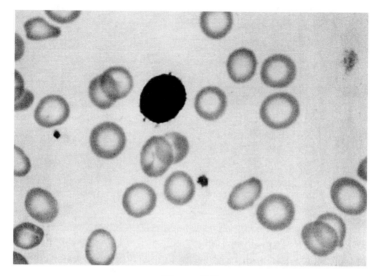

Figure 1.1

2. A finding inconsistent with iron deficiency would be

   A. decreased serum iron

   B. thrombocytosis

   C. a decreased plasma ferritin

   D. a decreased serum iron-binding capacity

   E. all of the above

3. Clinical conditions associated with the peripheral blood depicted in Figure 1.1 include

   A. GI hemorrhage

   B. intestinal malabsorption

   C. B12 deficiency

D. pregnancy

E. folate deficiency

Case Cluster (Questions 4–6):
Refer to Figure 1.2.

4. A 17-year-old Indonesian boy presents with a two-week history of fevers to 104° F and shaking chills. The peripheral blood smear is shown in Figure 1.2. This abnormality is consistent with

   A. a Döhle body

   B. intravascular *Bartonella bacilliformis*

   C. toxic granulations

   D. *Plasmodium falciparum*

   E. Philadelphia chromosome

Figure 1.2

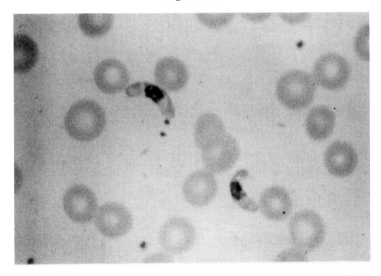

5. Non-drug-resistant first line treatment would likely include

   A. high-dose corticosteroids

   B. pyrimethamine-sulfadoxine

   C. broad-spectrum antibiotics

   D. chloroquine

   E. any of the above

6. Prophylaxis for malaria infections would **NOT** include

   A. weekly po Fansidar

   B. judicious use of bed netting and mosquito repellant

   C. weekly chemoprophylaxis with 500 mg chloroquine phosphate po

   D. avoidance of the tsetse fly Glossina

   E. mosquito repellant

Case Cluster (Questions 7–11):
Refer to Figure 1.3.

7. A 27-year-old sexually active white man presents with a one-day history of fever and right Achilles tendon pain. A purpuric skin lesion, seen in Figure 1.3, is present on the dorsum of his right hand. Diagnosis of this patient's illness often can be established by all **EXCEPT**

   A. culturing scrapings of the skin lesion

   B. culturing the blood

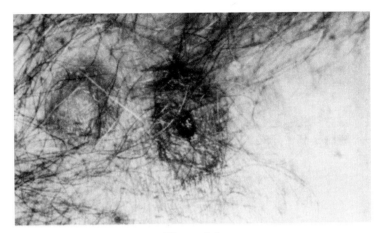

Figure 1.3

   C. right ankle joint aspiration and presence of intracellular gram-negative diplococci in the joint fluid

   D. direct fluorescent antibody staining of skin lesion scrapings

   E. punch biopsy and immediate direct visualization

8. Despite attempts to identify the etiology of the patient's illness, no diagnosis is made. Eight days after onset of his symptoms, the patient notes a tender, erythematous swelling of his left knee. Which of the following would be useful in diagnosing his condition?

   A. Aspiration of the left knee and culture of the joint fluid

   B. Pharyngeal culture

   C. Rectal culture

   D. MRI

   E. Blood cultures

9. A Gram's-stained slide obtained from the patient's anal canal reveals intracellular Gram-negative diplococci. Laboratory techniques that would help identify this agent as *N. gonorrhoeae* include all **EXCEPT**

   A. the ability to metabolize maltose

   B. a growth on Thayer-Martin agar

   C. a positive oxidase test

   D. the ability to metabolize glucose

   E. all of the above identify *N. gonorrhoeae*

10. Recommended therapy for disseminated gonococcemia includes all **EXCEPT**

    A. ceftriaxone 1gm IM or IV Q 24 hr

    B. ceftizoxime 1gm IV Q 8 hr

    C. aqueous penicillin G 10 million U/day IV for a minimum of 3 days, followed by ampicillin 500 mg 4 times a day Po for 10 days

    D. cefotaxime 1gm IV Q 8 hr

    E. procaine penicillin 10 million U-IM

11. All the following are true about female sexual contacts of the above patient who have contracted gonorrhea **EXCEPT**

    A. have approximately a 15% risk of developing pelvic inflammatory disease (PID)

    B. are often asymptomatic or minimally symptomatic

    C. may have up to a 5% incidence of infertility after recurrent PID

    D. may present with the clinical picture of cystitis

    E. are minimally symptomatic

Case Cluster (Questions 12–14):
Refer to Figure 1.4.

12. A 55-year-old black man presents with a two-month history of fatigue. His hematocrit is 34%. A smear of his peripheral blood is shown in Figure 1.4. These changes are consistent with

A. chronic blood loss

B. vitamin B12 deficiency or folate deficiency

C. sickle cell anemia

D. iron deficiency

E. acute blood loss

Figure 1.4

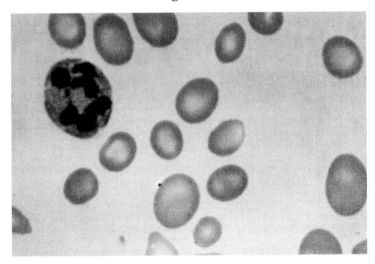

13. Further evaluation of this patient would likely include all of the following **EXCEPT**

    A. serum B12 levels

    B. bone marrow examination

    C. serum or red blood cell folate levels

    D. hemoglobin electrophoresis

    E. dietary history

14. The following are true about vitamin B12 absorption **EXCEPT**

    A. requires the presence of intrinsic factor

    B. may be decreased in patients with regional enteritis

    C. may be assessed by a Schilling test

    D. occurs primarily in duodenum

    E. involves the terminal ileum

Case Cluster (Questions 15–17):
Refer to Figure 1.5.

15. A 40-year-old man with a six-year history of intermittent bloody diarrhea undergoes the barium enema shown in Figure 1.5. GI complications of this disease include all **EXCEPT**

    A. toxic megacolon

    B. segmental involvement with granulomas

    C. colon carcinoma

    D. anal fistula

    E. colonic perforation

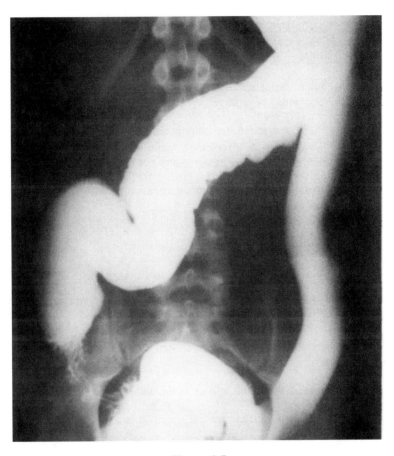

Figure 1.5

16. Which of the following statements pertaining to this disease is **NOT** true?

  A. Prophylactic colectomy is recommended in patients with universal colon involvement for longer than five years

  B. Ten percent of patients will have a prolonged remission after the first attack

  C. Sulfasalazine and 5-amino salicylate are generally effective in controlling early stages of the disease

  D. The appearance of the colonic mucosa in this disease may be mimicked by acute infectious colitis secondary to *Salmonella, Shigella, Campylobacter,* and amebiasis

  E. Surveillance colonoscopy is indicated

17. All are true about articular manifestations of inflammatory bowel disease (IBD) **EXCEPT**

  A. occur in approximately 25% of patients with IBD

  B. are often monoarticular or polyarticular involving peripheral joints

  C. ankylosing spondylitis associated with IBD parallels disease activity

  D. correlates with the activity of the underlying bowel disease

  E. tend to be self-limiting and not destructive

Case Cluster (Questions 18–19):
Refer to Figure 1.6.

18. Prior to treatment with methylprednisolone therapy, an intermediate strength 5 TU PPD is placed, which results in 15 mm of induration 48 hours later. The patient is unaware of any past exposure to tuberculosis and his chest radiograph is normal. Appropriate subsequent actions would include

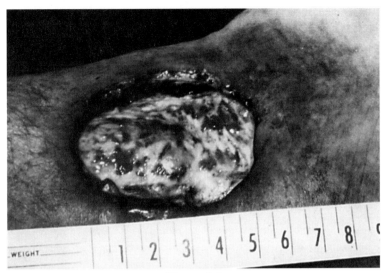

Figure 1.6

A. annual PPD (purified protein derivative)

B. serial chest radiograph every six months for two years

C. isoniazid 300 mg po qid for twelve months

D. rifampin 600 mg po qid for six months

E. boosted PPD (125 IU)

19. Major toxicity associated with the use of isoniazid includes all **EXCEPT**

A. hepatitis

B. influenza-like syndrome and thrombocytopenia

C. peripheral neuropathy

D. drug fever

E. thrombocytosis

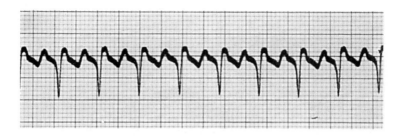

Figure 1.7

Case Cluster (Questions 20–21):
Refer to Figure 1.7.

20. The rhythm in Figure 1.7 may be associated with all **EXCEPT**

    A. organic heart disease

    B. acute respiratory failure

    C. pericarditis

    D. quinidine toxicity

    E. open heart surgery

21. Which of the following statements concerning this rhythm is false?

    A. Sinus rhythm is usually restored by carotid sinus massage

    B. The incidence of systemic emboli is less than that associated with atrial fibrillation

    C. DC cardioversion employing ≤ 50 joules is generally what is needed for conversion to sinus rhythm

    D. The ventricular rate may increase after administration of quinidine, disopyramide, or procainamide

    E. Disopyramide or procainamide would be helpful

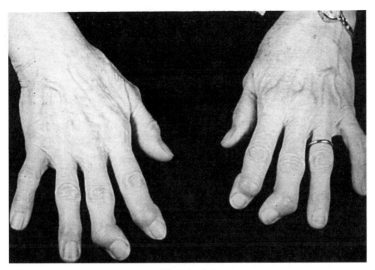

Figure 1.8

Case Cluster (Questions 22–23):
Refer to Figure 1.8.

22. Patients with the disorder manifested by the hands appearing in Figure 1.8 commonly demonstrate which of the following?

    A. Subcutaneous nodules on the extensor surfaces of the forearms in 20%-25% of patients

    B. Positive serum rheumatoid factor in 70% of patients

    C. Reduction in hemolytic complement levels in joint fluid to less than one third of serum levels

    D. Normal erythrocyte sedimentation rate (ESR) in most patients

    E. ANA positivity

23. Symptomatic patients with the disorder shown in Figure 1.8 may derive therapeutic benefit from

    A. aspirin or nonsteroidal antiinflammatory agents

    B. oral corticosteroids when symptoms are severe

    C. long periods of rest and disuse

    D. isotonic exercises involving affected joints, moving them through a full range of motion against progressively increasing resistance

    E. IV chelation therapy

Case Cluster (Questions 24–25):
Refer to Figure 1.9.

24. The abnormality in Figure 1.9 is commonly associated with all but which of the following disorders?

    A. Cystic fibrosis

    B. Renal insufficiency

    C. Hypertrophic osteoarthropathy

    D. Bronchiectasis

    E. Heavy smoking

25. Hypertrophic osteoarthropathy is characterized by all of the findings below **EXCEPT**

    A. pain and tenderness in the distal upper and lower extremities

    B. morning stiffness and polyarthritis involving the knees, ankles, wrists, elbows, and metacarpophalangeal joints

    C. frequent presence of subcutaneous nodules on the extensor surface of the forearm

    D. periosteal new bone formation in radiographs of distal parts of long bones

    E. periungal erythema

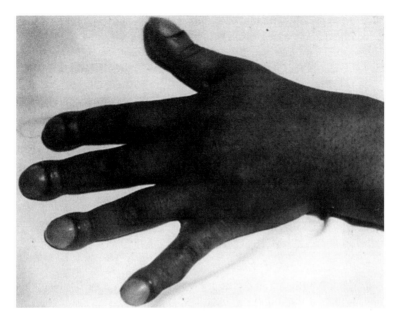

Figure 1.9

26. Michael, a 5-month-old that you have cared for since birth, is brought to your office by his mother for a routine visit. His mother reports that he is doing well, but she has been told by her mother that it's time to change Michael's feedings. She breastfeeds Michael every three to four hours during the day and occasionally feeds him in the middle of the night. Breast milk has been his sole source of nutrition. On physical examination, Michael is alert and playful. His weight and height are at the 25 percentile. She asks you for your advice regarding what to feed him now. Your advice to her is to

   A. begin rice cereal for its dietary source of iron

   B. continue on breast milk alone, adjusting the frequency as needed

   C. weigh Michael before and after feeding to assure Micheal is receiving adequate amounts of milk

   D. introduce finger foods such as biscuits and Cheerios

   E. begin strained or pureed meats to enhance protein intake as Michael continues to grow rapidly

27. A 5-year-old with fever, vomiting, and a rash is brought to the office. He has complained of a headache and sore throat. On exam he has circumoral pallor and hyperemic tonsils with a gray-white exudate. The entire pharynx is erythematous. His skin rash is papular and apparent in the axillae, groin, and antecubital fossae and is just appearing on the trunk. The most likely diagnosis is

A. scarlet fever

B. toxic shock syndrome

C. measles

D. Kawasaki disease

E. enteroviral exanthem

28. A 15-month-old arrives for a well child examination. He has had fever with each of his previous immunizations and the last immunization resulted in a local cellulitis requiring oral antibiotics. The most appropriate step to take at this time is

A. reassure the mother that her concern is well founded and the child should not receive any further immunizations; today you give no immunizations

B. reassure the mother that the problems her child has had are trivial and should not interfere with today's immunization; you give the age-appropriate immunizations

C. reassure the mother that fever is a common side effect and can be treated with antipyretics given before and after the immunization; you give acetaminophen, the age-appropriate immunizations, and directions for local care of the injection site

D. reassure the mother that her child is allergic to the immunizations and can be treated with chlorpheniramine; you administer the chlorpheniramine and the age-appropriate immunizations

E. reassure the mother that as her child has received most of the immunizations you can safely skip today's planned immunization; you give no immunizations

29. Matthew, an 8-year-old, returns to the office for follow-up of proteinuria. His initial urinalysis nine months ago was obtained as part of a pre-camp physical. He was, and continues to be, asymptomatic. Testing every three months, you have determined that the proteinuria is persistent. A test for orthostatic proteinuria revealed normal protein excretion in the supine position and increased urinary protein excretion when standing. His creatinine level is 0.7mg/dL. You inform the family that the prognosis for this problem includes

   A. likely maintenance of normal renal function although he will need regular follow-up

   B. gradual increase of proteinuria with development of a nephrotic syndrome

   C. rapid decline of renal function at the time of puberty but long-term risk of renal failure is low

   D. waxing and waning of renal function with a low likelihood of chronic renal failure

   E. gradual development of renal failure with likely need of dialysis by the age of 60

30. A 4-month-old male is brought to the clinic for evaluation of a scrotal mass which his mother noted during a recent diaper change. The findings on exam which would confirm a non-surgical diagnosis include

   A. a tender palpable mass associated with scrotal edema and overlying erythema

   B. a nontender palpable mass which increases in size while the infant is crying

   C. a nontender palpable mass which can be reduced with minimal effort

   D. a nontender, firm irregular mass

   E. a nontender mass which fails to change in size and transilluminates

31. A 3-year-old is brought to the office for evaluation of a bite. The historical information that suggests the highest likelihood of infection is

   A. the bite was inflicted by the family dog

   B. the child was bitten by a playmate while at daycare

   C. the bite was unwitnessed, but the child was seen playing with the next door neighbor's cat

   D. the child was bitten by a brown recluse spider

   E. the bite was inflicted by the family's pet monkey

32. A very distraught mother brings her teenage daughter into your office for evaluation of amenorrhea for the last three months. The 17-year-old girl previously had normal five-day menses every 28 days since menarche at 12 years of age. She denies sexual activity and refuses to have a pelvic exam. Important areas to assess in her history include all of the following **EXCEPT**

   A. physical activity and athletic training

   B. smoking history

   C. illicit drug use

   D. galactorrhea

   E. eating disorders or recent weight changes

33. Drugs or medications which can cause amenorrhea include all of the following **EXCEPT**

    A. oral contraceptives

    B. cyclophosphamide

    C. marijuana

    D. tricyclic antidepressants

    E. antibiotics

34. You are reviewing the pathology report on a recently performed sigmoid colon resection. Colorectal cancers described by Duke's classification include all of the following **EXCEPT**

    A. tumor limited to the submucosa

    B. tumor penetrating the bowel wall with no lymph node involvement

    C. presence of tumor within the bowel wall with lymph node involvement

    D. a highly differentiated tumor

    E. tumor metastatic to the liver

Case Cluster (Questions 35–36):

35. A 34-year-old woman presents to your office with abdominal pain of two weeks duration associated with grossly bloody diarrhea mixed with mucus. She has experienced several of these episodes over the past few months, and has noted a 12-pound weight loss over this period of time. You suspect inflammatory bowel disease. Which of the following statements regarding inflammatory bowel disease is incorrect?

    A. Both Crohn's disease and ulcerative colitis have an equal sex distribution

    B. Crohn's disease is three to five times more common in Jewish than non-Jewish populations

    C. Grossly bloody stools are common with Crohn's disease, but uncommon with ulcerative colitis

    D. Segmental full thickness inflammation of the bowel wall is the pathologic hallmark of Crohn's disease

    E. Continuous mucosal inflammation of the colon wall is the pathologic hallmark of ulcerative colitis

36. Examination of the patient reveals a tender left lower quadrant, and an examination of the stool reveals blood, mucus, and pus. She is afebrile. You have narrowed your diagnosis to ulcerative colitis. Which of the following is **NOT** a criterion for the differentiation of fulminating versus non-fulminating ulcerative colitis?

    A. Stool frequency greater than six per day

    B. Temperature greater than 38 degrees Celsius

    C. Erythrocyte sedimentation rate greater than 30 mm/hr

    D. Elevated hematocrit despite rehydration

    E. Tachycardia

37. A 25-year-old white male presents to the office with complaints of pain and swelling in both hands for approximately two months. He states that he is stiff each morning for approximately three hours. Examination reveals that the MCP joints and wrists of both hands are swollen, warm, tender, and have palpable synovial thickening. Hand X-rays show a periarticular decalcification. The most likely diagnosis in this patient is

A. degenerative arthritis

B. rheumatoid arthritis

C. systemic lupus erythematosus

D. psoriatic arthritis

E. gout

38. A 35-year-old black male with known sarcoidosis presents with polyuria as a manifestation of his disease. What is the likely pattern that will be observed?

A. Urine osmolality is high despite a low serum osmolality

B. Urine osmolality rises by greater than 9% following vasopressin injection in a water deprivation test

C. Urine osmolality is unaffected by vasopressin in a water deprivation test

D. Urine osmolality steadily increases during a water deprivation test in parallel with serum osmolality

E. A high urine osmolality is associated with a high serum glucose

39. A 52-year-old black man presents to the office with his third attack of acute gout in two months. Reasonable interventions at this time include the administration of colchicine or indomethacin plus

    A. starting allopurinol immediately

    B. starting probenecid immediately

    C. stop hydrochlorothiazide

    D. give oral prednisone

    E. give intraarticular steroids

40. A 42-year-old black man with known sickle cell disease presents with a two-month history of left hip pain. It is persistent over this time. He is afebrile and denies other systemic complaints and any history of trauma. The most likely diagnosis is

    A. sickle cell crisis

    B. trauma

    C. osteomyelitis

    D. degenerative arthritis

    E. aseptic necrosis of the hip

41. A 50-year-old white man presents with a several-year history of progressive increase in shoe size and enlargement of the tongue. Acromegaly is suspected. What is the most appropriate screening test for this condition?

    A. Random growth hormone level

    B. Glucose tolerance test

    C. MRI of the sella turcica

    D. Growth hormone response to thyrotropic releasing hormone (TRH)

    E. Growth hormone response to oral glucose load

42. A 45-year-old white man with mildly abnormal liver enzymes is found to have hepatitis C by screening. In counseling this patient, you can tell him that

   A. he has a 50% chance of developing chronic hepatitis or cirrhosis

   B. his sexual partner has a greater than 90% chance of acquiring the virus within one year

   C. interferon alpha has a greater than 50% cure rate

   D. alcohol consumption has little impact on developing chronic liver disease

   E. he may donate blood if his liver enzymes return to normal

Case Cluster (Questions 43–45):

43. A 45-year-old white man presents with a six-month history of fatigue. Physical examination is remarkable for a blood pressure of 160 /100 and multiple abdominal striae. Administration of 1 mg of dexamethasone at bedtime results in an 8 a.m. plasma cortisol of 10 mcg per deciliter (normal less than 5 mcg per deciliter). The next test to clarify the diagnosis is

   A. a plasma ACTH level

   B. low dose dexamethasone compression test (0.5 mg q 6 hours for 48 hours)

   C. metyrapone stimulation test

   D. cosyntropin stimulation test

   E. high dose dexamethasone suppression test (2.0 mg q 6 hours for 48 hours)

44. Subsequent testing in this patient reveals the failure of plasma cortisol to be suppressed to less than 50% of control value after 2 mg of dexamethasone every 6 hours for 48 hours. Of the diagnoses below, the most likely etiology of this patient's disorder would be

    A. pituitary microadenoma

    B. ectopic adrenal corticotrophic hormone production

    C. morbid obesity

    D. severe chronic depression

    E. chronic dilantin use

45. This patient is found to have a normal value for urine 17-OH ketosteroids, a normal CT scan of the abdomen, and a normal pituitary MRI. In this patient

    A. adrenal glands are likely to be atrophic

    B. adrenal carcinoma is very likely

    C. the most likely diagnosis is a small cell carcinoma of the lung

    D. abdominal exploration is indicated

    E. the abnormal dexamethasone suppression test was most likely a false positive

46. A 30-year-old white homosexual male presents with a six-week history of watery diarrhea, abdominal cramping, and weight loss. Of the infectious agents listed below, which would be the most likely cause?

    A. *Shigella*

    B. Cryptosporidiosis

C. *Salmonella*

D. *Campylobacter jejuni*

E. Toxogenic *E. coli*

47. A 58-year-old man is referred to you for evaluation because of a carotid bruit. Which of the following symptoms would suggest that this marks a symptomatic lesion?

A. Ipsilateral amaurosis fugax

B. Ipsilateral transient arm and leg weakness

C. Ipsilateral VIth nerve palsy

D. Recurrent, episodic vertigo

E. A dense, contralateral facial palsy involving the forehead

48. A 30-year-old woman presents with a blood pressure of 190/110. Initial laboratory evaluation reveals a serum potassium of 2.8. The next step in her evaluation would include

A. dexamethasone suppression test

B. urine screen for surreptitious diuretic use

C. renal arteriogram

D. plasma renin activity

E. urine prostaglandins

49. A 34-year-old man has the following test results on a serum lipid panel obtained after a 12-hour fast: total cholesterol = 300 mg per deciliter; high density lipoprotein (HDL) cholesterol = 40 mg per deciliter; triglycerides = 150 mg per deciliter. His low density lipoprotein (LDL) cholesterol can therefore be calculated as

    A. 110 mg per deciliter

    B. 260 mg per deciliter

    C. 150 mg per deciliter

    D. 230 mg per deciliter

    E. 190 mg per deciliter

50. You are performing a routine new patient physical examination on a 45-year-old asymptomatic black man in the office. On cardiac auscultation, you note paradoxical splitting of S2. This is most likely to be associated with

    A. mitral stenosis

    B. aortic insufficiency

    C. pulmonary hypertension

    D. left bundle branch block

    E. atrial septal defect

51. A 68-year-old Asian male returns to his physician's office reporting that he has lost all interest in his usual activities. He finds himself staring out his apartment window for hours at a time. He has recently retired from his business of twenty years. He is being treated by his physician for hypertension. The most appropriate next step for the physician to take is

    A. prescribe an antidepressant

    B. order a dexamethasone suppression test (DST)

    C. counsel the patient about the difficulties of retirement

    D. review his medication history

    E. refer to a psychiatrist for electroconvulsive therapy

52. A 46-year-old male with bipolar disorder has been followed in clinic for eight years. He has been taking lithium carbonate. Regular routine laboratory tests should include the following **EXCEPT**

    A. thyroid stimulating hormone (TSH) level

    B. dexamethasone suppression test (DST)

    C. serum creatinine level

    D. serum lithium level

    E. white blood cell count

Case Cluster (Questions 53–54):

53. A 37-year-old married white male who has been your patient for seven years presents in your office with a penile discharge. You diagnose gonorrhea and prescribe an antibiotic. He admits to you that he may have contracted the infection from a woman he met while out of town on a business trip. He knows that his wife, who is also your patient, is scheduled for her annual physical exam next week. He requests that you treat her, but not tell her why, suggesting that you could attribute the treatment to a urinary tract infection. The reasons **NOT** to comply with his request include all of the follow **EXCEPT**

    A. lying is morally condemned

    B. the doctor-patient relationship is fiduciary

    C. without disclosure, there can be no informed decisions

    D. disclosure can have more harmful than beneficial consequences

    E. one deception may necessitate another

54. Reasons for misrepresenting a diagnosis to a patient include all of the following **EXCEPT**

    A. Hippocrates urged physicians to do so

    B. physicians know what is best for the patient

    C. the patient does not want to be told

    D. misrepresentation could prevent serious harm to the patient

    E. the truth cannot be known

Case Cluster (Questions 55–57):

55. A 38-year-old female presents with complaints of a two-month history of episodic dizziness. She experiences distinct periods when she feels her heart pounding, tightness in her chest, tremulousness, and shortness of breath. Upon further questioning, some episodes have occurred when she is shopping. She has come to dread leaving the house. As you complete your medical history and physical examination and order appropriate laboratory tests, the **LEAST** likely diagnosis in your psychiatric differential would be

  A. social phobia

  B. panic disorder with agoraphobia

  C. anxiety disorder due to a general medical condition

  D. substance-induced anxiety disorder

  E. generalized anxiety disorder

56. Your workup is negative and you find no medical reasons for her symptoms. She is taking no other medications and denies taking any non-prescription drugs. Your working diagnosis is now panic disorder with agoraphobia. You would prescribe

  A. Paxil 20 mg qid

  B. Valium, 5 mg qid

  C. Haldol 2 mg qid

  D. Valium, 2 mg IV stat.

  E. Lithium, 300 mg tid

57. Two months later there is considerable improvement in her symptoms, but there is some residual anxiety under certain circumstances. Among options to consider, the most likely would be

  A. referral for psychoanalysis

  B. referral for cognitive-behavior therapy

  C. referral for electroconvulsive therapy

  D. see the patient every other week for supportive therapy

  E. change her medication

Case Cluster (Questions 58–63):

58. A 17-year-old male presents in your office with a chief complaint of "burning when I pee." He is sexually active, has a discharge from his penis and participated in passive anal intercourse. You have known this patient for the past ten years, but have not seen him in the last four years, except once for a sports physical about two years ago. Vital signs are normal. You begin by asking how he has been in general ("Fine"), and then proceed to take a more detailed history. The **LEAST** important fact would be

   A. how he is doing in school

   B. duration and degree of present symptoms

   C. medications taken for present illness

   D. past sexual partners

   E. details of kind of sexual activity

59. He appears to be in good general physical condition. You perform an exam, paying special attention to all of these. The **LEAST** important is

   A. fundoscopic exam

   B. rectal examination

   C. CVA tenderness

   D. examination of the testicles

   E. examination of the penis

60. You decide to order a number of laboratory tests. These include all **EXCEPT**

   A. scraping of penis surface

   B. gonorrhea culture of urethral discharge

   C. *Chlamydia* enzyme of penile discharge

   D. gram stain of urethral discharge

   E. HIV antibody test

61. You suspect GC urethritis. To confirm your diagnosis at this point, you would

   A. consult with a psychiatrist

   B. refer for a darkfield examination

   C. do a punch biopsy of the penile lesion

   D. review gram stain of urethral discharge

   E. do a Tzanck prep of scraping from penile lesion

62. The result of the test in question 61 was positive. As a result of all the information you have so far, you would do all **EXCEPT**

   A. treat with benzathine penicillin G 2.4 million units IM

   B. treat with aqueous procaine penicillin G 4.8 million units IM plus probenecid 1.0 gram by mouth, followed by tetracycline 500 mg qid for 1 week

   C. apply podophyllin in benzoin to the penis

   D. reschedule for a return visit and test of cure

   E. provide safer sex counseling

63. The patient returns four days after completion of therapy. He is free of symptoms. His present girlfriend has been evaluated and treated. His HIV test returns positive. Further management at this time includes all **EXCEPT**

A. PPD

B. RPR for syphilis if not already done

C. repeat test of cure culture

D. refer sexual partners for HIV testing

E. discuss prognosis

Case Cluster (Questions 64–69):

64. A 70-year-old man presented with a history of weakness, fatigue, dark stools, and increasing constipation of three-months' duration. He has had a long history of constipation, but it has gotten worse recently. He has also had episodes of diarrhea. He had an abdominal operation on a "big blood vessel" four years previously; he had a number of x-rays taken at that time and was told that his bowels were "okay for his age." Recently he feels tired all the time and cannot do the things he was able to do previously. He has lost ten pounds and has been taking vitamins and mineral supplements. Additional history of value in diagnosis includes all of the following **EXCEPT**

A. details of previous operation

B. results of bowel x-rays

C. sexual persuasion

D. nature of bowel movements

E. laxative use and medicines he is taking

65. Clinical evaluation should include all **EXCEPT**

A. abdominal distention and abdominal mass

B. splenomegaly

C. ascites

D. rectal examination

E. stool guaiac

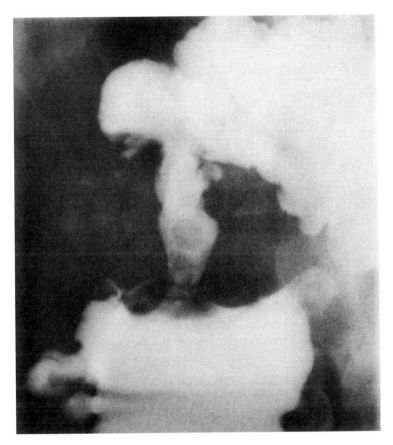

Figure 1.10

66. Initial investigations should include all **EXCEPT** (see Figure 1.10)

A. serum electrolytes

B. hemogram and liver profile

C. serum amylase and plain abdominal series

D. sigmoidoscopy

E. upper GI series and barium enema

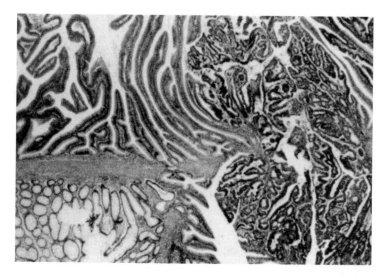

Figure 1.11

67. He is anemic and has an electrolyte abnormality. Additional studies and procedures required to confirm the diagnosis are (see Figure 1.11)

    A. upper endoscopy and biopsy

    B. electrolyte replacement

    C. serum carcinoembryonic antigen (CEA) levels

    D. mesenteric angiography and serum alpha-fetoprotein level

    E. parenteral vitamin K

68. Acceptable methods of treatment include

    A. bulk laxatives, antispasmodics, and reevaluation at frequent intervals

    B. primary resection and anastomosis or first-stage resection and colostomy and second-stage closure of colostomy

C. abdominoperineal resection

D. local excision

E. fulguration

69. Useful procedures in the follow-up care of this patient include all **EXCEPT**

A. sigmoidoscopy quarterly

B. colonoscopy annually

C. barium enema periodically

D. serum CEA levels

E. CT scan

Office

Answers and Discussion

1. **(E)** Hypochromic, microcytic blood cells can be seen in sideroblastic anemias, thalassemia, and anemia due to iron deficiency. Autoimmune hemolytic anemia is characterized by the presence of spherocytes in the peripheral blood, which appear as microcytic, hyperchromic cells with evidence of hemolysis. (**Ref. 1**, pp. 315–316, 1743)

2. **(D)** Decreased serum iron and an increased serum iron-binding capacity are characteristic of iron deficiency. Reduced plasma ferritin accurately reflects deficient iron stores. The platelet count can be increased or normal in iron deficiency anemia. (**Ref. 1**, pp. 1723–1724)

3. **(C)** Iron deficiency results from decreased intake, increased requirements, decreased absorption, or blood loss. Pregnancy increases daily iron requirements threefold. GI blood loss is the most important cause of iron deficiency in adult males, while menstrual blood loss is the most common cause in women of child-bearing age. Malabsorption, especially of the duodenum and jejunum, may result in iron deficiency. B12 and folate deficiencies are present with megaloblastic anemias. (**Ref. 1**, pp. 1723–1724, 1726–1727)

4. **(D)** The abnormality depicted in Figure 1.2 is a *Plasmodium falciparum* gametocyte. Bartonellosis is an infection with *Bar-*

tonella bacilliformis, a disease limited to certain valleys in the Andes mountains. Unlike these infections of red blood cells, Döhle bodies and toxic granulations are abnormalities of neutrophils found in infections and other toxic states. (**Ref. 1,** pp. 887–895)

5. **(D)** Treatment for all types of acute malaria, except drug-resistant falciparum, can be achieved with chloroquine. Due to the emergence of drug-resistant falciparum in Southeast Asia and South America, acute infections of falciparum require the use of combination therapy, including quinine, pyrimethamine, and the use of the sulfonamides or sulfones. High-dose corticosteroids and broad-spectrum antibiotics have not been found to be of benefit in the treatment of acute malaria. (**Ref. 1,** pp. 893–895)

6. **(D)** Chloroquine is effective in preventing the primary episodes of *P. vivax* and *P. ovale.* In areas endemic for chloroquine-resistant *P. falciparum,* weekly Fansidar (pyrimethamine, 25 mg and sulfadoxine, 500 mg) should be used concurrently. The vector, the Anopheles mosquito, should be avoided by netting, repellents, and proper clothing. The tsetse fly is important in the transmission of African trypanosomiasis, not malaria. (**Ref. 2,** p. 891)

7. **(A)** The patient's history is classic for disseminated gonococcal disease. Blood cultures and direct fluorescent antibody staining of skin lesion scrapings can establish the diagnosis in over 50% of cases during the early stage of dissemination. Joint fluid is usually sterile but can show diplococci during the initial stage of disseminated gonococcemia. The diagnosis is more readily established by immunofluorescent staining of skin lesions rather than by culture of the scrapings. (**Ref. 1,** p. 647)

8. **(E)** During the later stages of disseminated gonococcemia, the synovial culture is positive in at least 50% of cases. Pharyngeal and rectal cultures will establish the diagnosis in some additional cases. Blood cultures are rarely positive in the later stage. MRI is unlikely to be helpful. (**Ref. 1,** p. 647)

9. **(A)** *Neisseria* strains grow on the selective Thayer-Martin medium, and both *N. meningitidis* and *N. gonorrhoeae* yield positive oxidase reactions. *N. gonorrhoeae* metabolizes glucose but not maltose. **(Ref. 1,** p. 648)

10. **(C)** These two regimens are effective in disseminated gonococcemia. One-time-only procaine penicillin and 7 days of oral tetracycline are effective in uncomplicated anogenital infections in heterosexuals, but not in disseminated gonococcemia. **(Ref. 1,** p. 648)

11. **(C)** The endocervix and urethra, at a rate of almost 80% to 90%, are the most commonly involved sites of infection. Approximately one half of women with gonorrhea are minimally symptomatic or asymptomatic. Presenting symptoms include vaginal discharge, hemorrhage, or may mimic cystitis caused by Gram-negative bacilli. The major complication of PID is infertility, estimated to be 15% after one episode, and about 50% after three episodes. **(Ref. 1,** p. 647)

12. **(B)** The peripheral blood smear is significant for macrocytic oval red blood cells (macroovalocytes) and a polymorphonuclear leukocyte with a hypersegmented nucleus. These changes are seen in the megaloblastic anemias secondary to vitamin B12 and folate deficiencies. Chronic blood loss and iron deficiency are characterized by microcytic, hypochromic red cell morphology. Sickle cell anemia is manifested by both normocytic and sickled cells on examination of the peripheral blood. **(Ref. 1,** pp. 1726–1727)

13. **(D)** Because the patient has a macrocytic anemia, evaluation would include both vitamin B12 and folate levels. A bone marrow examination can be helpful. Hemoglobin electrophoresis would not be indicated in this patient with a macrocytic anemia. **(Ref. 1,** p. 1730)

14. **(D)** A deficiency of intrinsic factor, or diseases involving the terminal ileum (regional enteritis), the site of vitamin B12 absorp-

tion, can result in vitamin B12 deficiency. The Schilling test helps to delineate the etiology of vitamin B12 deficiency. (**Ref. 1,** pp. 1730–1731)

15. **(B)** The clinical history and loss of haustra with narrowing of the left colon suggest ulcerative colitis. GI complications include all of the answers listed; in addition to colonic perforation, one can see colonic stricture, rectal prolapse, and massive colonic hemorrhage. Segmental involvement with granulomas are the hallmarks of Crohn's disease. (**Ref. 1,** p. 1407)

16. **(A)** In the past some authorities have advocated prophylactic colectomy to prevent colon cancer in patients with ulcerative colitis of more than ten-years' duration. The present option is careful surveillance colonoscopy to obtain multiple sequential biopsies assessing for mucosal dysplasia. Anticholinergic drugs and opiates are generally not effective in controlling diarrhea in the setting of severe colitis and actually may contribute to the development of toxic megacolon. Sulfasalazine and 5-amino salicylate PO or PR are mainstays of treatment of mild diseases. Infectious colitis may mimic ulcerative colitis. (**Ref. 1,** p. 1413)

17. **(C)** Articular manifestations are present in approximately 25% of patients with IBD over the course of their disease. A monarticular or polyarticular form commonly involves knees, ankles, and wrists and parallels the activity of the bowel disease. It is usually self-limiting and joint destruction is not seen. The central arthritis (ankylosing spondylitis) is not related to the course of the underlying bowel disease. (**Ref. 1,** p. 1413)

18. **(C)** Serial chest radiographs are not cost-effective in the follow-up of patients with positive PPDs. As the patient under discussion is likely to receive chronic, high-dose steroid therapy, treatment with isoniazid for one year is indicated. Rifampin is indicated for one year for a new PPD converter if the patient has been exposed to a source case infected with tubercle bacilli documented to be resistant to isoniazid. Once a patient demon-

strates a positive reaction to PPD, repeat PPD testing is contraindicated as this may result in severe local tissue necrosis. (**Ref. 1,** p. 715)

19. (**B**) There is 3% to 5% incidence of hepatitis in patients taking isoniazid and rifampin. Induction of P-450 cytochrome system by drugs such as alcohol or barbiturates predisposes to isoniazid hepatitis. The hepatitis usually resolves with prompt discontinuation of the drug. A reversible peripheral neuropathy, associated with isoniazid use, can be prevented or treated with pyridoxine. Drug fever can also occur. Influenza-like syndrome and thrombocytopenia are seen with rifampin, not isoniazid. (**Ref. 1,** p. 715)

20. (**D**) Atrial flutter occurs in patients with organic heart disease, acute respiratory failure, pericarditis, and open heart surgery. Quinidine toxicity is most frequently manifested as bradyarrhythmias, conduction disturbances, and ventricular arrhythmias. (**Ref. 1,** p. 1023)

21. (**A**) In contrast to atrial fibrillation, the atria contract during atrial flutter, which may account for the lesser incidence of systemic emboli associated with atrial flutter. Because they slow the rate of atrial contraction and enhance AV-node conduction, type I antiarrhythmics (quinidine, disopyramide, and procainamide) may increase the ventricular response rate in patients with atrial flutter, converting 2:1 atrioventricular conduction to 1:1 conduction; this may be prevented by coadministration of digoxin, propranolol, or verapamil. Carotid sinus massage rarely converts atrial flutter to sinus rhythm. DC cardioversion with low energies (≤ 50 joules) will frequently convert atrial flutter to sinus rhythm. (**Ref. 1,** p. 1023)

22. (**D**) Figure 1.8 demonstrates bony enlargement and spur formation along the distal interphalangeal joints (Heberden's nodes) and proximal interphalangeal joints (Bouchard's nodes) of the fingers characteristic of osteoarthritis. The ESR is normal in most patients. RF is negative. (**Ref. 1,** pp. 1688–1697)

23. **(A)** Therapy for osteoarthritis includes aspirin or nonsteroidal antiinflammatory agents to relieve pain and decrease inflammation. Corticosteroids are usually ineffective in improving symptoms from osteoarthritis. Isometric exercises are more likely to maintain muscle function and strength without aggravating joint symptoms than are isotonic exercises against resistance. Long periods of rest and disuse can lead to muscle contractions. (**Ref. 1**, p. 1697)

24. **(B)** Clubbing may be a finding in each of these disorders except renal insufficiency. (**Ref. 1**, pp. 1196, 1705–1706, 1145)

25. **(C)** Hypertrophic osteoarthropathy may include all of the manifestations listed in A, B, D, and E. While this disorder may sometimes be mistaken for rheumatoid arthritis, it is not associated with rheumatoid nodule formation. (**Ref. 1**, p. 1705)

26. **(A)** Breast milk, in sufficient quantity, can supply sufficient calories for growth in infants under 12 months of age. However, iron, required for prevention of anemia, should be supplemented by four to six months of age when the infant's body stores from birth are depleting. Rice cereal not only contains iron, but is the most hypoallergenic grain. Weighing of infants before and after breastfeeding should be discouraged. (**Ref. 6**, pp. 1010–1011)

27. **(A)** Scarlet fever is caused by an infection by streptococci that produce pyrogenic exotoxins. Children present with hyperemic tonsils that may be covered with an exudate. The oropharynx, including the tongue, is inflamed. The exanthem is erythematous and punctate or papular. It appears first in the axillae, groin, and neck but can generalize over the entire body. Toxic shock syndrome is associated with toxin-producing *S. aureus* and results in a diffuse erythematous macular rash associated with headache, fever, vomiting, and diarrhea. Measles is characterized by conjunctivitis, photophobia, and cough. Koplik spots are usually seen in the throat. Kawasaki disease presents with a rash, conjunctival involvement, and a persistent high

fever. Enteroviral exanthems are usually papular and often associated with mild respiratory and gastrointestinal symptoms. (**Ref. 5,** pp. 751–752)

28. **(C)** Benefits and risks of immunization must be discussed with families prior to their administration. While it is not unusual for fever or a mild to moderate local reaction including redness, soreness, and swelling to occur following an immunization, they are not a contraindication to immunization. Precautions should be taken if the temperature reaches a level of 40.5 degrees C or higher within 48 hours of a DTP. True contraindications, as identified by the CDC, include anaphylactic reactions to a vaccine, development of an encephalopathy within seven days of a DTP, known immunodeficiency including infection with HIV in the patient or household contact, and pregnancy (for MMR and oral polio). The mother's concerns are real and if trivialized may result in failure to complete the immunization series. A 15-month-old will most likely have received DTP, HIB, hepatitis, and polio vaccines, but would not yet have received the MMR (**Ref. 6,** pp. 3–38)

29. **(A)** Proteinuria in three consecutive samples can be found in up to 2% of girls and 0.5% of boys but frequently resolves spontaneously. For children with persistent proteinuria, orthostatic proteinuria is the etiology in over 60% of cases. Orthostatic proteinuria, defined as elevated protein excretion only while in the upright position, does not appear to be of clinical significance. Biopsies from patients with orthostatic proteinuria are generally normal and there appears to be no long-term effect on renal function. However, long-term studies in children are lacking and follow-up should be provided. (**Ref. 6,** pp. 3–38)

30. **(E)** Scrotal masses can be caused by such problems as inguinal hernias, hydroceles, testicular torsion, epididymitis, and neoplasms. Testicular torsion, resulting in a tender mass with edema and erythema, is a surgical emergency. Nontender masses which increase with crying and are reducible are suggestive of hernias. Hernias also require surgical repair to prevent the possible complication of incarceration of abdominal contents. Firm, irregular

masses in the scrotum are suggestive of a malignancy and require surgical exploration. Non-communicating hydroceles often resolve spontaneously and do not require surgical intervention unless they become painful. (**Ref. 6,** pp. 58–60)

31. **(B)** Millions of injuries due to bites are evaluated each year. The majority of mammalian bites are due to dogs (80%) while smaller percentages are due to cats and humans. The risk of infection depends on the type of mammal that bites. Only 4% of dog bites become infected, while 35% of cat bites and 50% of monkey bites result in infection. Nearly all human bites that puncture skin, especially the hand, become infected and require treatment. Brown recluse spider bites result in local inflammation and ulceration due to the venom introduced but are rarely associated with infection. (**Ref. 5,** pp. 2027–2030)

32. **(B)** This patient has amenorrhea as defined by a lack of menses for total of at least three of the previous menstrual intervals. A careful history should evaluate for the following causes: strenuous physical activity or athletic training, eating disorders or weight fluctuations, family or social stress, previous or current health problems, sexual activity, pregnancy, normal secondary sex characteristics including a previous functioning menstrual tract. Substance abuse, especially marijuana and amphetamines, can cause amenorrhea. (**Ref. 9,** p. 404)

33. **(E)** Although all the other medications can cause amenorrhea, it has not been associated with antibiotics. (**Ref. 9,** p. 404)

34. **(D)** The Duke's classification of colorectal tumors is based on tumor extension, not histology. While tumor size does not predict the likelihood of metastasis or survival, tumor extent as described by the Duke's classification predicts prognosis reasonably well. In Duke's classification, stage A tumors are limited to the mucosa and submucosa. Stage B tumors are confined to, or penetrate, the bowel wall without nodal metastasis. Stage C and D tumors involve spread to local lymph nodes or to other organs, respectively. (**Ref. 18,** p. 1217)

35. (C) The inflammatory bowel disease is divided into two types, Crohn's disease and ulcerative colitis. Crohn's disease is defined pathologically by segmental full thickness inflammation of the bowel wall. Crohn's occurs more commonly in the Jewish population, and between the ages of 15 and 40 years old. Patients with both Crohn's disease and ulcerative colitis can present with abdominal pain, diarrhea, and weight loss. However, grossly bloody stools are the hallmark of ulcerative colitis. Ulcerative colitis is defined pathologically by continuous mucosal inflammation of the colon wall. It occurs more commonly in whites who reside in industrialized nations. A family history is present in 15% to 20% of cases. (**Ref. 12,** pp. 1653–1654)

36. (D) Parameters suggestive of fulminant ulcerative colitis include all except item D. Aside from those listed, other criteria include a hematocrit less than 30% after rehydration, weight loss in excess of 10% of premorbid weight, serum albumin concentration less than 3 gm/dl, failure of normally successful treatment regimens, and failure of a five- to seven-day course of intensive outpatient therapy. (**Ref. 12,** p. 1654)

37. (B) This patient meets five of the seven criteria for rheumatoid arthritis. He presents with morning stiffness greater than one hour, arthritis involving three or more joint areas, arthritis of the hand joints, symmetric arthritis, and radiograph changes consistent with rheumatoid arthritis. Degenerative arthritis tends to involve more distal joints in the fingers and have less evidence of inflammation. Systemic lupus erythematosus can involve the hands symmetrically, as in this case, but it usually does not have evidence of periarticular bone resorption. Psoriatic arthritis tends to affect the DIP joints as well. Gout is typically asymmetric and is characterized by acute flares of monoarticular arthritis. (**Ref. 1,** p. 1653)

38. (B) Sarcoidosis can manifest as centrally mediated diabetes insipidus. When osmolality rises greater than 9% following vasopressin injection in a water deprivation test, this indicates that diabetes insipidus is present and is likely of central origin. When the urine osmolality is high, despite a low serum osmolality, it is indicative of the syndrome of inappropriate antidiuretic hormone secretion (SIADH). When urine osmolality is unaffected by vasopressin in a water deprivation test, this indicates a renal cause of diabetes insipidus. When urine osmolality increases during a water deprivation test in parallel with serum osmolality, it suggests that the primary etiology is most likely primary polydipsia. Finally, a high serum glucose associated with a high urine osmolality is indicative of diabetes mellitus. (**Ref. 1,** pp. 1924–1927)

39. **(C)** Allopurinol and probenecid can prevent recurrent attacks of gout and ultimately are indicated in patients such as this; however, all signs of acute inflammation should have disappeared before starting these medications because the acute drop in uric acid concentration may prolong or precipate an acute attack. Prednisone is almost never used in the treatment of gout; however, intraarticular steroids may be indicated, if an acute attack of gout is not responding to the traditional first line of therapy, or if colchicine and indomethacin are contraindicated. Hydrochlorothiazide can cause increases in serum uric acid and in a patient with recurrent attacks it is very reasonable to stop this medication. (**Ref. 1,** pp. 2085–2086)

40. **(E)** The significant features of this case are the age of the patient and the fact that this pain is persistent and unremitting. Sickle cell crisis is typically episodic and rarely lasts more than three to five days. Osteomyelitis could give persistent pain, particularly in an older sickle cell patient; however, this is usually associated with at least low-grade fevers. Degenerative arthritis could certainly give isolated hip pain, but would be unusual in a 42-year-old individual without underlying joint destruction such as aseptic necrosis or trauma. There is no history of trauma to this hip, making this less likely. Aseptic necrosis is quite common in sickle cell patients as they get older and should be suspected in any patient over the age of 30 who presents with persistent joint pain. (**Ref. 1,** p. 1737)

41. **(E)** The growth hormone response to a glucose load should be suppressed to less than 2 micrograms per liter. Greater than this suggests abnormal growth hormone secretion. Measurement of so-

matomedin C may also be indicative of acromegaly. Random growth hormone levels are unreliable and vary throughout the day. Glucose tolerance tests are often impaired, but this is not a specific test. An MRI of the sella turcica is abnormal in most patients with acromegaly; however, this is usually not indicated until laboratory screening suggests that acromegaly may be present. Eighty per cent of pituitary tumors have an increase in growth hormone with the administration of TRH; but this is not sensitive enough to act as a screening test. (**Ref. 1,** pp. 1900–1901)

42. **(A)** Hepatitis C causes little acute illness and has an insidious progress, but unfortunately has at least a 50% chance of progressing to chronic hepatitis or cirrhosis. Epidemiology shows us that sexual transmission occurs but is not likely. Interferon alpha is one of the few drugs that has an impact on the progress of hepatitis C. Approximately 50% of patients will respond to initial treatment of intraferon alpha, but approximately half of these relapse when the drug is stopped. The presence of other insults to the liver, in particular alcohol, can increase the likelihood that a patient will go on to develop chronic liver disease. (**Ref. 1,** pp. 1463, 1480)

43. **(B)** The formal diagnosis of Cushing's syndrome is the demonstration of the inability to suppress 24-hour urine cortisone, plasma cortisone, or 17-hydroxy steroid excretion following low-dose dexamethasone suppression (0.5 mg q 6 hours × 46 hours). Plasma ACTH levels are useful in distinguishing the cause of the syndrome by illustrating ACTH dependent vs. independent hypercortisolism. The metyrapone test can be used instead of high-dose dexamethasone suppression to elucidate ectopic or ACTH-independent cortisol secretion. The cosyntropin stimulation test is used for the diagnosis of adrenal insufficiency. (**Ref. 1,** pp. 1962–1963)

44. **(B)** The high-dose dexamethasone suppression test should suppress secretion triggered by pituitary microadenoma. Failure to suppress suggests there is ectopic ACTH production or there is an autonomously functioning adrenal mass, such as an adrenal malignancy. Morbid obesity can trigger hypercortisolism which is

usually suppressed on the high-dose test. Similarly, severe chronic depression can be associated with abnormal elevations of cortisone and, again, this is usually readily suppressed with a high-dose dexamethasone suppression test. (**Ref. 1,** pp. 1952–1953)

45. (C) The abnormal high-dose dexamethasone suppression test narrowed the differential diagnosis down to ectopic adrenal corticotrophic hormone (ACTH) production or adrenal carcinoma. Adrenal carcinomas are usually associated with elevated urinary 17-OH ketosteroids and are typically seen on a CT scan of the abdomen. Occasionally, a large pituitary mass can lead to a relatively nonsuppressable plasma cortisol as well. However, this is ruled out by the normal pituitary MRI. This leaves ectopic adrenal corticotrophic hormone (ACTH) secretion as the most likely diagnosis. The most common cause of this would be small cell carcinoma of the lung. (**Ref. 1,** pp. 1952–1953)

46. (B) A white homosexual male raises the question of AIDS-related diarrhea. In this population, cryptosporidiosis and isospora bella are some of the more common etiologies. Even if this patient does not have AIDS, this appears to be a chronic diarrhea and does not have many acute features. *Shigella, Salmonella, Campylobacter jejuni,* and toxogenic *E. coli* all cause acute disease, which is relatively short-lived and associated with intensive abdominal cramping and occasional hematochezia. (**Ref. 1,** pp. 675, 678, 680, 912)

47. (A) The carotid circulation feeds the parietal lobes and the ophthalmic artery. An embolus from a lesion in the carotid artery would cause blockage in the ophthalmic artery on the same side, leading to ipsilateral amaurosis fugax. An embolus going to the middle cerebral artery on the same side would cause transient arm and leg weakness on the contralateral side. Fixed nerve palsies are most commonly found in diseases such as diabetes mellitus, but would be associated with the posterior circulation as opposed to the carotid circulation. Recurrent episodic vertigo without focal neurologic signs is rarely due to cerebral vascular disease. However, vertigo would be a vertebral basilar symptom as opposed to a carotid distribution syndrome. A dense facial palsy involving the forehead indicates a peripheral facial nerve lesion such as Bell's palsy. (**Ref. 1,** p. 2239)

48. **(D)** The most common cause of hypokalemia associated with hypertension is hyperaldosteronism. Accordingly the initial work-up is geared toward identifying the presence of this disorder. The first step is typically a plasma renin activity. If elevated, one then pursues a saline load test with measurement of plasma aldosterone. The dexamethasone suppression test screens for Cushing's syndrome. Renal artery arteriograms could reveal renal artery stenosis which should be considered in any young woman because of the possibility of fibromuscular dysplasia. Renal artery stenosis can also lead to hypokalemia, although hyperaldosteronism would be much more common. Urine prostaglandins can be a marker for Bartter's syndrome, but this disorder is not typically seen with significant hypertension. (**Ref. 1,** p. 1996)

49. **(D)** The formula for calculating LDL cholesterol is: total cholesterol − HDL − (triglycerides/5). This calculates to 230 mg per deciliter in this individual. This formula is valid as long as triglycerides remain below 400 mg per deciliter. The triglyceride level divided by 5 correlates with the level of VLDL cholesterol, since most triglycerides are contained within the VLDL lipoprotein. When the triglyceride level climbs above 400 mg/dl, chylomicrons are present and the estimation of the VLDL no longer holds. (**Ref. 1,** p. 1111)

50. **(D)** Paradoxic splitting of S2 occurs when P2 precedes A2 such that the split is maximized in expiration and decreases in inspiration. The most common causes are left bundle branch block, delayed excitation of the left ventricle such as after a right ventricular ectopic, and severe mechanical outflow obstruction as in aortic stenosis. Atrial septal defect may cause a fixed split in S2. Pulmonary hypertension will cause a loud P2. (**Ref. 1,** p. 951)

51. **(D)** Many antihypertensive medications (including propranolol and drugs containing reserpine) have been implicated in causing depression. Changing the antihypertensive medication will often alleviate the depressive symptoms without resorting to an antidepressant or other active treatment. The DST was a popular screening test for depression in the early 1980's but more recently, its utility has been called into question. It is also premature to order the test before obtaining the medication history. Counseling and referral should not precede a thorough assessment of the etiology of the depression. (**Ref. 10,** p. 570)

52. (**B**)   The DST has no role in the follow up monitoring of lithium carbonate maintenance. Lithium has a thyroid-suppressing effect. It is also known to cause a leukocytosis. Reports of possible kidney damage with long-term use necessitate following kidney function with serum creatinine levels. Generally lithium reaches a steady state level with little subsequent change unless there are conditions that interfere with this equilibrium. Potassium sparing diuretics or dehydration may result in an increased serum lithium level. This is due to reabsorption in the kidney where it is normally excreted. (**Ref. 10,** pp. 964–965)

53. (**D**)   Actually, if this statement were true it would argue for complying with the husband's request. In fact disclosure usually has more beneficial than harmful consequences. In addition to permitting informed decisions, it facilitates treatment compliance and mobilization of support from friends and family, avoids incorrect speculation, and helps the patient focus on treatment options. (**Ref. 18,** pp. 57–63)

54. (**B**)   This paternalistic stance was commonplace several decades ago. This has changed to a respect for an individual's autonomy. The last three reasons have been given as justification for withholding a grave prognosis or diagnosis from a patient. Hippocrates did, in fact, urge doctors to conceal "most things from the patient while you are attending him." (**Ref. 18,** pp. 58–59)

55. (**E**)   The essential feature of generalized anxiety disorder is excessive worry or anxiety more days than not, lasting at least six

months. Her symptoms do not meet the time criteria. At this point, you have not ruled out medical or medicinal sources of her anxiety. The increasing isolation could be due to social phobia or agoraphobia. (**Ref. 16,** pp. 60–61)

56. (A) Benzodiazepines must be used at much higher than usual doses and only specific triazolobenzodiazapines such as alprazolam or clonazepam appear to have antipanic effects. There is no indication for intravenous injection. Virtually all antidepressants seem to have antipanic properties. Tricyclic Antidepressants, Selective Serotonin Reuptake Inhibitors, and Monoamine Oxidase Inhibitors have demonstrated efficacy. Antipsychotics such as Haldol and antimanic medication such as lithium are not indicated here. (**Ref. 11,** pp. 450–460)

57. (B) Cognitive behavioral therapy has been shown to be beneficial in panic disorders, especially when incorporating exposure techniques. Psychoanalysis is a long-term process that may not be indicated if the patient is seeking primarily symptom relief. ECT is not indicated for this condition and supportive therapy is less effective. Changing medication is premature at this point. (**Ref. 11,** pp. 456–460)

58. (A) Although important, of those listed, school performance would have the least impact on making a diagnosis at this point. Many people feel that any contact with an adolescent demands a special history, abbreviated HEADS (home, education & employment, activities, drugs, and sexuality). A quick review of these areas with appropriate questioning will give a good sense of how the young person is coping with adolescence. Answer A is considered incorrect because of the form the question takes, which allows the teen to answer with one word, accomplishing nothing. "What are you good (bad) at in school?" is a better way to elicit information. Open-ended questions are better. Onset of symptoms is always important as is timing of any medication taken, which may affect culture results.

A complete sexual history is very important. It should include starting with the question: "Have you had sexual relations with anyone? Do you have sex with men, women, or both?" This is a nonjudgmental, straightforward way of getting the needed information. One then proceeds to ask about a current steady sexual partner and how many partners in the last month(s). Next one must identify sites at risk. In our patient, all three sites are at risk. Specific questions are often needed to determine this. "Did you put your penis in his (her) mouth? Did you put your penis in his rectum? Did he put his penis in your mouth? Did he put his penis in your rectum? Were condoms used, and if so did they break?" So a good sexual history determines: (1) if the individual is having sexual relationships; (2) sexual orientation; (3) if there is a current steady partner; (4) number of recent partners; (5) sites at risk; (6) safer sex practices; and (7) any concerns about sexual dysfunction. (**Ref. 1,** pp. 26–27)

59. **(B)** In the physical exam, one would be concerned about thorough examination of the genitalia and rectum. Pharyngeal gonorrhea (GC) is often unremarkable on exam. Funduscopic exam in this situation is pointless. CVA tenderness may be a sign of pyelonephritis in the presence of urinary tract infection. (**Ref. 1,** pp. 646–647)

60. **(A)** The critical laboratory tests are GC cultures of all sites at risk, and a gram stain of the urethral discharge. An enzyme *chlamydia* test would be beneficial. It is not essential for making a diagnosis of nongonococcal urethritis (NGU). Laboratory tests such as CBC, electrolytes, chest x-ray, and urine culture are not indicated. Urinalysis is not likely to be helpful in view of the urethral discharge. Surface scraping of the penis is unnecessary. In view of his high-risk behaviors, especially passive anal intercourse without a condom, a human immunodeficiency virus (HIV) antibody test should be done. (**Ref. 1,** p. 760)

61. **(D)** Further management at this time is to look at the gram stain for the presence of gram-negative intracellular diplococci. Punch biopsy is not indicated. One could not argue with doing an RPR test for syphilis, but it will not help with immediate management, and ideally we will treat the patient with a regimen that is effec-

tive against incubating syphilis. There are no lesions suggestive of syphilis (darkfield not indicated) or herpes (Tzanck prep not needed). (**Ref. 1,** pp. 644–650)

62. **(B)**   We have a clear diagnosis of GC urethritis. Because of frequent co-existence of *chlamydia,* GC is now double-treated with a regimen effective against both. If he were not at risk rectally, the treatment would be ampicillin 3.5 g PO plus probenecid 1g PO, now, followed by tetracycline 500 mg qid for one week. Because of the potential of rectal GC, he should be treated with a regimen effective for that. Podophyllin is treatment for venereal warts, but none were found. With increasing numbers of GC resistance nationwide, a follow-up test of cure should be arranged. Sexual partners need to be informed, evaluated, and epi treated. Safer sex counseling is highly appropriate. (**Ref. 1,** pp. 648–650)

63. **(C)**   Follow-up management in this case is critical. Most centers that do HIV antibody testing will actually perform three tests before calling the result positive. These include an ELISA test that is positive, and a repeat ELISA test that is also positive. We are thus faced with a young, healthy, sexually active, adolescent, bisexual who is HIV-antibody positive. Many of these cases are in people in their twenties, which means they probably had initial contact with the virus in their teens. AIDS is the end-stage disease of infection with HIV. The Walter Reed staging system is an effective way to emphasize that infection with this virus is a continuum. What causes progression from one stage to another is unknown, as is the time it may take for such progression. Best estimates are that 50% or more of infected individuals will develop full-blown AIDS within five to ten years of becoming HIV-antibody positive. Discussing prognosis is appropriate.

The management of this young man at this time includes a PPD (the increase in tuberculosis nationwide is in part due to HIV infection), and an RPR (syphilis may act differently in people who are HIV-antibody positive: there may be a more rapid progression of syphilis, and more intense follow-up is needed). Sexual partners need to be referred to determine their HIV-antibody status. This is especially true in bisexuals in order to prevent perinatal transmission.

Referral to an "AIDS specialist" may be appropriate if available, though initial management can certainly be done by most practicing physicians. Review of what the patient needs to be alert to (lymphadenopathy, fatigue, fevers, weight loss, oral candidiasis) is appropriate, as is a discussion of how to prevent further transmission, including safer sex practices: avoiding donation of blood, sperm, or body organs; not sharing toothbrushes, razors, or other items that might be contaminated by blood; and cleaning surfaces contaminated with blood with household bleach (1:10 dilution with water). Many communities have developed programs for the "worried well," and referral to such an agency may be helpful. No repeat test of cure culture is necessary. (**Ref. 1,** pp. 645–649, 1570)

64. **(C)** The presentation of this 70-year-old man with increasing constipation, weakness, dark stools, and fatigue should lead to a strong suspicion of cancer of the left colon. The patient does have a long history of constipation, but the important feature is the change in the bowel habits in the recent past. The episodes of diarrhea are probably related to fecal impaction and consequent mucus secretion. The weight loss also suggests a diagnosis of malignancy of the colon.

   The family history is useful to make sure that there are no other contributory factors but is not valuable in diagnosis. Most patients with a history of familial polyposis develop their cancer at a very early age, and so it is unlikely that is a contributing factor in this man. The nature of bleeding with colonic cancer is such to produce melena. On the other hand, massive colorectal bleeding is seen in diverticular disease, but the nature of his bleeding does not indicate that it is due to the same. The increasing usage of laxatives indicates that his colonic lumen was perhaps being compromised, and he was developing some degree of intestinal obstruction. Older individuals take a large number of medicines and it is important to check if the patient is on any medicines that are likely to produce bleeding (e.g., potassium supplements, antiarthritic medications). (**Ref. 14,** pp. 1025–1026, 1259–1272)

65. **(B)** Patients with left colon strictures may have abdominal distention due to partial intestinal obstruction. This patient has un-

dergone an aortoiliac anastomosis in the past and may have had a segment of ischemic colitis. Therefore, in addition to strictures due to diverticular disease and malignancy, one should consider ischemic colitis as a cause. Left colon lesions are seldom palpable as a mass, although a mass may be palpable in a number of patients with right colon cancer. Once a suspicion of colonic cancer is entertained, one should evaluate the patient for extent of the disease in terms of liver metastases and ascites. This patient did not demonstrate these findings. Rectal examination and examination of the stool for guaiac is an absolute necessity in any patient with these symptoms. In this patient, the lesion is too far above (30 cm from the anus) to be felt with examining finger, but the stool was positive for guaiac, indicating some bleeding. Splenomegaly does not. (**Ref. 14,** pp. 1025–1026, 1198–1200, 1262, 1467)

66. (**C**) In patients with a colonic lesion plus an electrolyte abnormality such as hyponatremia, hypokalemia, or hypochloremia, a suspicion of a villous adenoma should be raised. The fact that this patient had diarrhea, off and on, should increase the suspicion. The hemogram shows that the patient is anemic; this could be due partly to actual blood loss and partly to a dilutional effect. Serum amylase was not indicated in this patient because acute pancreatic disease was not suspected. The liver profile is a useful investigation not only to determine liver function but also to evaluate for any evidence of metastatic disease (indicated by abnormal liver enzymes, hyperbilirubinemia, etc.) A plain abdominal series in this patient is useless. Most radiologists obtain a plain film of the abdomen prior to doing an upper GI series or a barium enema. Therefore, as a separate study it has no value. A sigmoidoscopy is absolutely indicated; however, in this patient the lesion was more proximal and was not useful. An OCG was not indicated since biliary disease was not being seriously considered. An upper GI series is useful in evaluation because the patient does have bleeding per rectum. This study would exclude proximal causes of melena, such as cancer of the stomach, bleeding varices, or a duodenal ulcer. Occasionally, small bowel polyps account for bleeding particularly on the left side, and, therefore, an IVP is indicated. It is preferable to do this on the same day as doing the barium enema but prior to the enema because once the barium is introduced to the colon, it may cause problems in interpretation of the IVP. The most useful of these tests is the barium enema. (**Ref. 14,** pp. 1025–1026, 1173, 1262)

67. **(C)** The further studies are to determine the cause of the stricture more precisely and to plan the management. An upper endoscopy and biopsy are, therefore, not indicated on the basis of the previous studies. Colonoscopy and biopsy are indicated for a lesion at this level. In further management, the patient should have a replacement of electrolytes to correct the abnormalities. In addition, a serum CEA level should be obtained as a baseline because it would prove useful in subsequent management. Serum alpha-fetoprotein levels are useful in the evaluation of hepatic tumors, not colon cancers. Mesenteric angiography is not indicated in this patient. The degree of bleeding is a slow, steady one and is not significantly brisk to be useful in localization of the bleeding site. Further, in this patient at the time of the presumed aneurysm, the inferior mesenteric artery was probably ligated, and, therefore, there is no indication for it. The patient is anemic; preoperatively, he should be transfused so that he can tolerate anesthesia. Similarly, he should be started on parenteral hyperalimentation because of his previous weight loss and age and because he was probably nutritionally depleted. There is no need for parenteral vitamin K because the patient has no evidence of any obstructive jaundice. At this stage, consideration should be given to elective resection of the colonic lesion and the bowel should be prepared. Bowel preparation includes mechanical bowel preparation, both from below and also by using liquid diets and laxatives orally. In addition to mechanical bowel preparation, the patient should be given oral nonabsorbable antibiotics such as neomycin- and erythromycin-based preparations to reduce the bacterial flora and the infective complications of bowel resection. (**Ref. 14,** pp. 1025–1026, 1271–1278)

68. **(B)** The ideal procedure for treatment of the lesions shown is a primary resection including a good length of bowel proximally and distally. Such length should include at least 10 cm on each side, and a primary anastomosis can be performed. However, if at the time of resection there were other factors such as tension at the anastomosis or risk of leakage, one could do a resection of the

tumor and a proximal colostomy with the idea of going back into the abdomen for a second-stage closure of the colostomy. That is an acceptable alternative. Since the patient does not have any acute emergency such as an obstruction, the three-stage procedure was often considered. Abdominoperineal resection is not indicated because even by removing 10 cm distally, the patient would still have decent length of rectum and an anastomosis can be performed. Bulk laxatives, antispasmodics, and other conservative measures are useful in the management of diverticular disease, and they are not of value when the patient has a stricture. Similarly, local excision or fulguration is inadequate. Fulguration by itself might result in perforation of the colon in this lesion and sepsis and death. (**Ref. 14,** pp. 1025–1026, 1271–1278)

69. (**E**) Presuming that the patient has had no metastatic disease in the liver or in the peritoneal cavity and has undergone a primary resection with anastomosis, he should be carefully followed periodically for evidence of recurrence. Sigmoidoscopy is simple and should be performed at quarterly intervals. The anastomosis itself probably would be in the reach of the sigmoidoscopy and the area should be examined for any suture line or other recurrence. Since the patient has had colon cancer, he should be examined colonoscopically annually and barium enema is an acceptable alternative. A chest x-ray is not a high priority since colon cancer most often spreads to the liver and it is only in the late stages that there are any lung lesions. There is no value in doing serum alpha-feto-protein levels or urinary 5-HIAA levels in this patient. On the other hand, if after the operation, the patient's serum CEA levels were within the normal range and subsequently they were elevated, it would indicate a recurrence or metastatic disease. Therefore, CEA levels should be measured. Quarterly CT scans of the abdomen are not justified. When one is looking for metastatic disease in the liver, ultrasonography or a liver function test would be equally useful. A CT scan is only indicated if there is some suspicion of metastatic disease based on other tests. A routine CT scan is economically unjustified.

This patient is an interesting problem because he has a colonic lesion that could have been due to diverticulitis, ischemic colitis, or cancer. In the postoperative management, the value of sigmoidoscopy and CEA levels cannot be overemphasized. (**Ref. 14,** pp. 1025–1026, 1271–1278)

2

Hospital

DIRECTIONS (Questions 1–44): Each of the numbered items or incomplete statements in this chapter is followed by answers or completions of the statement. Select the **ONE** lettered answer or completion that is **BEST** in each case.

---

1. A 6-month-old infant is admitted in January for wheezing and respiratory distress. He developed increasing work of breathing and tachypnea and now is audibly wheezing. His physical examination and radiographic studies confirm the likely diagnosis of bronchiolitis. His older sister has had rhinorrhea and a cough for several days. The optimal specimen for definitive diagnosis of the most likely etiologic agent is

   A. nasopharyngeal swab

   B. tracheal aspirate

   C. nasopharyngeal washings

   D. throat swab

   E. blood for viral titers

2. You are called to the nursery to see a newborn with respiratory distress and cyanosis. On exam you hear a soft holosystolic murmur. The child is breathing at 80/minute. Oxygen saturation while in room air is 68% by pulse oximetry and does not change with the administration of 100% oxygen. The chest radiograph appears relatively normal. The most appropriate next step is

   A. transfer to a Level III nursery

   B. obtain an electrocardiogram

   C. begin administration of 100% oxygen

   D. begin administration of prostaglandin E_1

   E. call cardiology for an emergency consultation

3. You are caring for a 3-year-old with pneumonia, dehydration, and persistent hypoxemia requiring hospitalization. She has had little oral intake and continues to require oxygen. Her nurse just noted several vesicular lesions on her scalp and trunk. You discover that your patient was exposed to a child with varicella in her daycare setting two weeks ago. The appropriate next step is

   A. discharge her with careful instructions on the management of pneumonia and dehydration

   B. place her in an isolation room with a filtered air system

   C. determine at-risk patients and health care workers by obtaining their previous history

   D. begin acyclovir therapy to decrease the severity of the disease

   E. administer varicella-zoster-immune globulin to your patient and patients in adjacent rooms

4. An 18-month-old with Tetralogy of Fallot has been admitted for evaluation of increasing instances of cyanotic episodes. You are called to her bed during one of these episodes. She initially became tachypneic and restless, then became cyanotic. The appropriate next step is

   A. administration of subcutaneous morphine

   B. providing oxygen through a bag/mask device

   C. administration of beta adrenergic agents

   D. correction of acidosis with sodium bicarbonate

   E. placement of infant on the abdomen in the knee-chest position

5. A 10-year-old black male has been admitted for treatment of sickle cell pain crisis. He is currently receiving morphine for control of his extremity pain with reasonable results. His heart rate is 115, respiratory rate is 32/min and oxygen saturation is 85% in room air. He is afebrile. Physical examination reveals mild intercostal retractions, a grade II/VI systolic murmur at the left sternal border, a soft abdomen with diminished bowel sounds, and improvement in his extremity pain. The most likely etiology for his current problem is

   A. acute splenic sequestration

   B. anemia causing decreased oxygen carrying capacity

   C. subacute bacterial endocarditis

   D. acute chest syndrome

   E. pneumonia

6. A 12-year-old was admitted to the hospital after being struck by an automobile. His physical examination revealed a right hemotympanum, chest wall abrasions, liver laceration, and fractures of the right femur and right radius. He received appropriate therapy including morphine for pain control. Several days after admission he developed a fever and altered mental status. The most appropriate next step is

    A. perform a ventilation/perfusion scan to evaluate for a pulmonary embolus from his fractured femur

    B. obtain serum ammonium and liver function tests to evaluate for liver failure with hepatic encephalopathy

    C. perform a lumbar puncture to evaluate for meningitis

    D. obtain a blood culture and begin antibiotics for possible sepsis

    E. obtain a chest radiograph to evaluate for atelectasis secondary to hypoventilation

7. You have been caring for a 16-year-old with osteosarcoma of the right tibia with metastases present at diagnosis. She underwent above-the-knee amputation and chemotherapy. Despite this, her metastases are increasing in size. She was admitted for treatment of respiratory distress and has slowly been deteriorating. Her parents have been hesitant to directly address the fact that she is dying, but realized that this question was coming. During your visit with her she states: "I am dying, aren't I?" The appropriate next step is

    A. acknowledge the question but defer the discussion with her until her parents are available

    B. acknowledge that we will all die some day, but hopefully it will be in the future

    C. ignore the question and quickly change the subject, as she is a minor and discussions must take place with her parents

    D. emphasize that her acute problem is what you are treating and discuss your plans

    E. acknowledge the question and begin a discussion about her concerns, contacting the parents when possible

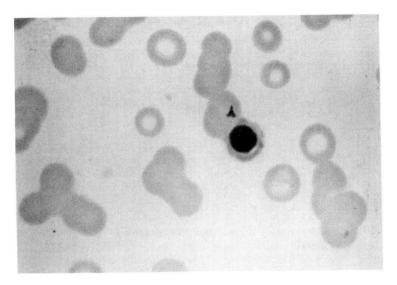

Figure 2.1

Case Cluster (Questions 8–10):
Refer to Figure 2.1.

8. A 65-year-old white man presents with complaints of fatigue and lower back pain for three months. His hematocrit is noted to be 30. The indices are normocytic, normochromic. Lytic lesions are seen in the skull films. Serum and urine immunoglobulins are elevated and his peripheral blood is shown in Figure 2.1. The abnormalities shown are consistent with

   A. alcoholic liver disease

   B. multiple myeloma

   C. vitamin B12 deficiency

   D. folate deficiency

   E. chronic iron deficiency anemia

9. The patient develops nausea, vomiting, constipation, and mental confusion. The most likely etiology in this patient is

    A. hyperglycemia

    B. hyperuricemia

    C. hypokalemia

    D. hypoglycemia

    E. hypercalcemia

10. Initial treatment for the condition described might include all EXCEPT

    A. IV normal saline

    B. loop diuretic

    C. Ca^{+2} binding resin

    D. biphosphates

    E. EDTA

Case Cluster (Questions 11–13):
Refer to Figure 2.2.

11. A 58-year-old white man presents with a two-week history of gingival bleeding. A slide of his peripheral blood is shown in Figure 2.2. Conditions associated with microangiopathic hemolytic anemias and decreased platelet counts (as shown in Figure 2.2) include all of the following EXCEPT

    A. malignant neoplasm

    B. prosthetic valves

    C. retained fetus and aminotic fluid

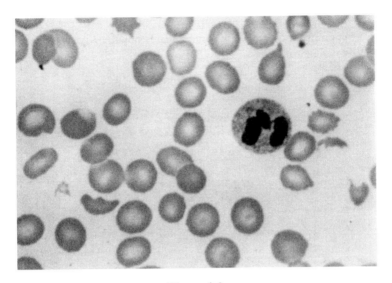

Figure 2.2

D. sepsis

E. vascular malformation and thrombosis

12. Laboratory testing revealed the following values concerning the patient:
    Prothrombin time 16 sec (normal 10–12 sec)
    Plasma fibrinogen 120 mg/dL (normal 160–415 mg/dL)
    Hematocrit 33% (normal 45%–55%)
    Platelet count 100.000/mm^3 (normal 150,000–400,000/mm^3)
    These values are consistent with

    A. early hemochromatosis

    B. surreptitious heparin use

    C. disseminated intravascular coagulation (DIC)

    D. isolated vitamin K deficiency

    E. all of the above

13. Further examination of the peripheral blood reveals the presence of promyelocytes with hypergranular cytoplasm. Appropriate therapy might include all **EXCEPT**

A. induction therapy for acute promyelocytic leukemia

B. treatment of acidosis if present

C. appropriate therapy for infection or acidosis

D. prevention of infection with face masks, etc.

E. high-dose steroids

Case Cluster (Questions 14–16):
Refer to Figure 2.3.

Figure 2.3

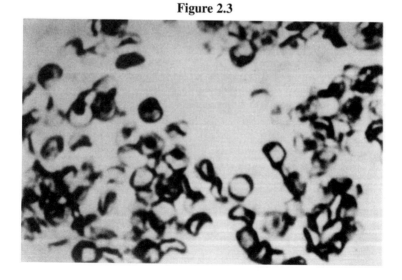

14. A 30-year-old white male homosexual who had practiced unsafe sex for five years presents with a two-month history of fever and weight loss. A biopsy of a skin lesion is interpreted as Kaposi's sarcoma. A diagnosis of acquired immunodeficiency syndrome (AIDS) is made. Persons **NOT** at high risk to develop AIDS include

    A. IV drug users

    B. household contacts of AIDS patients

    C. patients with hemophilia A

    D. medical personnel exposed to AIDS patients via deep intermuscular injections

    E. individuals practicing unsafe sex

15. Two months after diagnosis, the patient notes a nonproductive cough and slight dyspnea on exertion. Chest x-ray reveals bilateral interstitial infiltrates. Likely etiologies include all **EXCEPT**

    A. pneumococcal pneumonia

    B. cytomegalovirus pneumonia

    C. nonspecific interstitial pneumonitis

    D. *Pneumocystis carinii* pneumonia

    E. all four are likely etiologies

16. Due to a failure to respond to broad spectrum antibiotics, the patient underwent open lung biopsy. Staining with Gomori methenamine silver reveals large numbers of the organism shown in Figure 2.3. Treatment options include all **EXCEPT**

    A. clindamycin and primaquine

    B. parenteral pentamidine

    C. IV acyclovir

    D. oral trimethoprim-sulfamethoxazole

    E. IV trimethoprim-sulfamethoxazole

Case Cluster (Questions 17–19):
Refer to Figure 2.4.

Figure 2.4

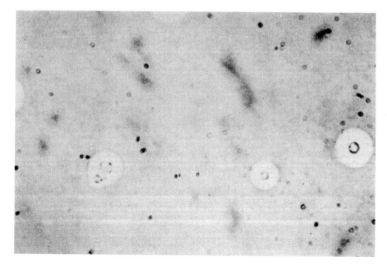

17. A 40-year-old white man with diffuse histiocytic lymphoma develops nausea, headache, and blurred vision. Lumbar puncture reveals CSF with

> Protein 85 mg/100 mL (normal < 40 mg/100 mL)
> Glucose 35 mg/100 mL: serum glucose 130 mg/100 mL
> (normal CSF glucose: serum glucose ratio > 60%)
> Leukocytes 80 cells/mm^3: 86% lymphocytes, 15% neutrophils
> (normal < 5 cells/mm^3: with 100% lymphocytes)
> Red blood cells 0

All the following are possible diagnoses **EXCEPT**

    A. tuberculous meningitis

    B. aseptic meningitis

    C. fungal meningitis

    D. cerebral aneurysm

    E. parameters are consistent with all of them

18. Examination of the spinal fluid of this patient reveals the abnormality seen in Figure 2.4. Another study likely to diagnose this condition includes

    A. CT scan of the brain

    B. blood culture

    C. technetium brain scan

    D. latex agglutination cryptococcal antigen of CSF

    E. viral culture of CSF

19. Complications commonly associated with therapy for this disorder include

    A. hypokalemia

    B. colitis

    C. hepatic insufficiency

    D. peripheral neuropathy

    E. anemia

Case Cluster (Questions 20–22):
Refer to Figure 2.5.

20. A 3-year-old boy presents with a several-hour history of fever, altered mental status, and the rash shown in Figure 2.5. The differential diagnosis would include

Figure 2.5

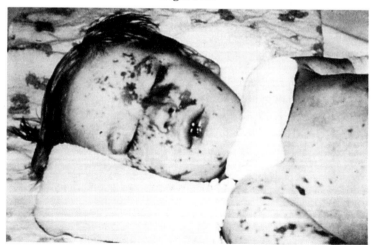

A. Kawasaki disease

B. meningococcemia with meningitis

C. Tackiasu's aortitis

D. bronchopulmonary dysplasia

E. Lyme disease

21. The diagnosis of meningococcal disease may be established by all **EXCEPT**

A. spinal fluid culture

B. culture of petechial scrapings

C. counterimmunoelectrophoresis (latex agglutination)

D. culture of the nasopharynx

E. blood culture

22. Prophylaxis for meningococcal disease

A. should be given to all intimate contacts

B. can be achieved by rifampin 600 mg/day for 2 days

C. can be achieved by minocycline 100 mg every 6 hours

D. can be achieved by penicillin VK 500 mg every 12 hrs for 5 days

E. all of the above

23. A patient in the intensive care unit develops a fever, elevated white blood cell count, and jaundice. His suspected diagnosis is acalculous cholecystitis. Factors that predispose to acalculous cholecystitis include all of the following **EXCEPT**

    A. diabetes mellitus

    B. hepatitis

    C. recent major operative procedure

    D. burns

    E. trauma

24. You are talking with the family of a head-injured patient admitted to the ICU under your care. The patient has suffered a traumatic subdural hematoma. Which of the following represents incorrect information regarding acute subdural hematoma?

    A. Subdural hematoma implies a blood collection located between the dura and the arachnoid membranes

    B. Subdural hematoma is caused by arterial bleeding

    C. Acute subdural hematoma is more common following head injury than epidural hematoma, but much less common than post-traumatic subarachnoid hemorrhage

    D. Acute subdural hematoma has a 60% to 80% mortality rate

    E. Damage to the brain parenchyma is often associated with acute subdural hematoma

25. A 78-year-old male with longstanding rheumatoid arthritis treated with hydroxychloroquine and aspirin is admitted to the hospital with fever. He is found to have splenomegaly. A CBC shows a white blood cell count of 3,000 with a differential of 10 neutrophils, 85 lymphocytes, 4 eosinophils, and 1 basophil. His hemoglobin is 11.9 and reticulocyte count is 1.4%. A likely diagnosis is

    A. acute leukemia

    B. drug reaction to hydroxychloroquine

    C. pneumococcal sepsis

    D. Felty's syndrome

    E. Coomb's mediated hemolytic anemia

Case Cluster (Questions 26–27):

26. A 56-year-old white man with a prior splenectomy is admitted to the intensive care unit for pneumococcal sepsis. Physical examination is unremarkable except for a question of a delayed relaxation phase of the deep tendon reflexes in the ankle. Serum T-3 is decreased. The differential diagnosis would include hypothyroidism and

    A. subacute thyroiditis

    B. increased concentration of thyroxin binding globulin

    C. euthyroid sick syndrome

    D. Grave's disease

    E. euthyroid Hashimoto's thyroiditis

27. For the scenario in the previous question, the most appropriate test to differentiate the likely causes of the low serum T-3 would be

    A. a radionuclide uptake scan

    B. a serum TSH

    C. anti-thyroid antibodies

    D. thyroid globulin level

    E. sedimentation rate

28. A 45-year-old white male patient with acute renal failure has been found to have a serum potassium of 6.8 milliequivalents per liter. What further diagnostic studies need to be done emergently in order to assess this patient?

    A. Serum blood urea nitrogen (BUN) and creatinine

    B. Serum magnesium

    C. Serum calcium

    D. Urine electrolytes

    E. ECG

29. An 86-year-old woman presents with obtundation. A family member states that she has been ill for approximately one week. Laboratory reveals a BUN of 110 mg/dl and a creatinine of 9 mg/dl. A calculated fractional excretion of sodium (FeNa) is less than 1.0%. A renal ultrasound is normal. The likely diagnosis is

    A. acute tubular necrosis

    B. prerenal azotemia

    C. bladder neck obstruction

D. glomerular nephritis

E. interstitial nephritis

Case Cluster (Questions 30–31):

30. A 24-year-old white man presents with a four-week history of an enlarged right cervical lymph node. He denied a history of fever, sweats, or weight loss, but had noted a generalized itching for two weeks. Examination revealed a 3 cm. cervical lymph node. The remainder of the physical exam was normal. Lymph node biopsy revealed nodular sclerosing Hodgkin's disease. Subsequent workup included a normal chest and abdominal CT scans, normal lymphangiogram, and a normal laparotomy. In the Ann Arbor classification for Hodgkin's disease, his disease would be

    A. Stage Ia

    B. Stage Ib

    C. Stage IIa

    D. Stage IIb

    E. Stage III

31. For the patient in the preceding question, the treatment of choice is

    A. subtotal nodal irradiation

    B. total nodal irradiation

    C. chemotherapy

    D. chemotherapy plus local irradiation

    E. excision of the node with localized irradiation

32. A 54-year-old white man is about to undergo coronary artery by-pass surgery. This surgery will prolong his survival if

   A. he has unstable angina

   B. he has left main coronary disease and impaired left ventricu-lar function

   C. he has right coronary artery disease and a recent subendocar-dial infarction

   D. he has stable angina with a 90% stenosis of the circumflex artery

   E. he has atrial fibrillation

Case Cluster (Questions 33–34):

33. You are covering the psychiatric service when you are called to the hospital's internal medicine service because a patient is insisting on leaving the hospital even though his laboratory tests indicate an increasing anion gap. The intern wants you to declare the patient incompetent so that the team can continue appropriate treatment. Your options include all of the following **EXCEPT**

   A. speak to the patient and make a mental status examination

   B. speak to the patient and assess for competency

   C. speak to the house staff about their concerns

   D. speak to the house staff and discuss criteria for involuntary commitment

   E. speak to the patient to check his understanding of the situation

34. You believe your patient requires additional hospitalization to adequately treat her condition. The patient's utilization reviewer denies further hospitalization. The **LEAST** indicated option is to

A. immediately discharge the patient

B. discuss the situation with the patient, including your recommendations

C. appeal the decision

D. advocate on behalf of the patient

E. continue to treat the patient in the hospital

Case Cluster (Questions 35–39):

35. A 32-year-old professional athlete has been admitted for surgical correction of a knee injury. The surgical procedure proceeds uneventfully. On the second hospital day, the patient has a generalized tonic-clonic seizure. There has been no prior history of seizure disorder. Possible causes of the seizure include all of the following **EXCEPT**

A. CNS neoplasms

B. alcohol withdrawal

C. hypernatremia

D. head injuries

E. CNS infections

36. If we assume that the seizure is related to alcohol withdrawal, appropriate responses include all of the following **EXCEPT**

    A. initate carbamazepine (Tegretol) 800 mg per day

    B. initiate an organic workup to identify the etiology of the seizure

    C. observe for other signs of withdrawal

    D. placing a padded tongue blade at the head of the bed

    E. order chlordiazepoxide (Librium) IM

37. The symptoms of alcohol withdrawal delirium or delirium tremens (DTs) include all of the following **EXCEPT**

    A. tactile or visual hallucinations

    B. hyperexcitability

    C. lethargy

    D. tachycardia

    E. hypothermia

38. The best treatment for DTs is

    A. physical restraint

    B. prevention utilizing benzodiazepines

    C. fluid restriction

    D. low carbohydrate diet

    E. isolation

39. Wernicke's syndrome and Korsakoff's syndrome are related for the following reason

    A. both are chronic conditions

    B. both are irreversible conditions

    C. both are related to thiamine deficiency

    D. Korsakoff's syndrome often progresses to Wernicke's syndrome

    E. both syndromes include blackouts

Case Cluster (Questions 40–44):

40. A 65-year-old obese white man was admitted with lower abdominal colicky pain of three-days' duration. The pain was in the suprapubic area and in the left lower quadrant. In the past one year he had similar pain on three occasions, but it usually resolved in a day or two. He also complained of increasing constipation and episodes of diarrhea for the last six months. He has not vomited but feels nauseated and has abdominal distention. He has not passed any stool or gas per rectum for 24 hours but has noted that he has "passed gas" along with urine. On admission his vital signs were T 100.6° F, P 96, BP 150/90 Wi. Required additional clinical information includes all **EXCEPT**

    A. rectal bleeding

    B. weight loss

    C. alcohol intake

    D. abdominal tenderness

    E. rectal exam

41. Initial workup should include all **EXCEPT**

    A. CBC

    B. urine culture

    C. stool culture

    D. plain abdominal series

    E. ultrasound examination of abdomen

42. Management of this patient at this stage will include

    A. IV fluids and parenteral antibiotics

    B. oral neomycin and erythromycin

    C. bulk laxative

    D. cecostomy

    E. colostomy

43. Subsequent studies to delineate any of this patient's lesions should include all **EXCEPT**

    A. barium enema

    B. CT scan

    C. cystoscopy

    D. cystogram

    E. urethrogram

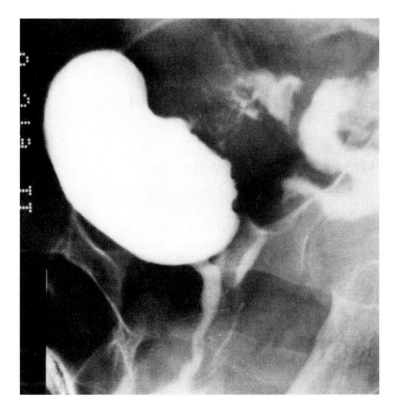

Figure 2.6

44. Results of the evaluation include Figure 2.6. Treatment of this lesion is accomplished by

A. primary resection of colon, repair of bladder, and suprapubic drainage

B. colostomy and partial cystectomy

C. bladder drainage and parenteral hyperalimentation

D. transurethral prostatectomy, proximal colostomy, and hyperalimentation

E. transurethal prostatectomy

Hospital

Answers and Discussion

1. **(C)** The most frequent etiologic agent for a young infant with bronchiolitis in the winter months is the Respiratory Syncytial Virus (RSV). Although both cultures and immunofluorescent may be positive using specimens obtained via nasopharyngeal swab or throat swab, a culture obtained from a nasopharyngeal washing is optimal for definitive diagnosis. A tracheal aspirate is unnecessary and invasive. (**Ref. 5,** pp. 905–906)

2. **(D)** A cyanotic newborn whose oxygen saturation fails to improve on 100% oxygen should be considered to have a congenital heart lesion where there is obstruction to outflow of blood from the right ventricle resulting in intracardiac shunting from right to left. The child described here is symptomatic and requires immediate intervention. Administration of prostaglandin E1 results in an opening of the ductus arteriosus and allows enhanced pulmonary blood flow and improvement in oxygenation. Obtaining an ECG, cardiology consult, and transfer to a higher intensity nursery are all appropriate but should not prevent the institution of PGE1 to prevent hypoxic-ischemic damage. (**Ref. 6,** pp. 1493–1497)

3. **(B)** Transmission of varicella is via close person-to-person contact or via airborne spread and is possible for several days prior to the onset of the rash. Patients who develop varicella while hospi-

talized put noninfected caretakers and immunocompromised patients at risk. If varicella exposure is known prior to hospitalization, placement in a room with a filtered air system will minimize exposure of others. Once varicella lesions occur, placement in a similar room is necessary to minimize further risk. Varicella-zoster-immune globulin should be administered to patients cared for in the same room or to those immunocompromised patients exposed. Oral acyclovir has not altered the course of the disease in otherwise healthy patients. More than 90% of adults with a negative history for varicella have titers that support previous infection. (**Ref. 6,** pp. 684–686)

4. **(E)** "Tet spells" are episodes of paroxysmal dyspnea and cyanosis. Treatment of these episodes includes a series of interventions beginning with positioning the child on her abdomen in a knee-chest posture. This increases the systemic vascular resistance and affects the return of blood to the right side of the heart. Oxygen supplementation is often provided, but is of little assistance during the episode of decreased pulmonary blood flow. Prolonged attacks may be treated by administration of morphine and/or sodium bicarbonate to treat the acidosis which develops. Increasing the systemic vascular resistance with vasopressors such as methoxamine or phenylephrine is done when other treatment fails but beta adrenergic agents are contraindicated. (**Ref. 6,** pp. 1497–1502)

5. **(D)** Sickle cell anemia affects 1 in 600 African-Americans and results in frequent episodes of vaso-occlusive crises, infection, and long-term complications such as stroke and renal failure. Acute chest syndrome, resulting from pulmonary infarction, presents with hypoxemia and respiratory distress. It may be associated with pneumonitis or microscopic evidence of fat emboli. Acute chest syndrome may be difficult to differentiate from pneumonitis in the febrile patient. Splenic sequestration occurs in infants and young children, presenting with signs of circulatory compromise and a massively enlarged spleen. Anemia is universal in children with sickle cell disease and can result in decreased oxygen carrying capacity. However, symptoms of anemia include tachycardia with a normal oxygen saturation. Children with sickle cell disease

are not at increased risk of subacute bacterial endocarditis. SBE presents with a new murmur and fever but is usually not associated with hypoxemia. (**Ref. 5,** pp. 1396–1400, 1345)

6. (**C**)   Most basilar skull fractures close spontaneously within 72 hours of injury. However, a basilar skull fracture results in open communication between the meningeal space and the nasopharynx or middle ear. Fever and altered level of consciousness in a child with a known basilar skull fracture require evaluation of the CSF. Pulmonary emboli are infrequent in children, but can occur from fractures. Presenting signs and symptoms include respiratory distress and hypoxemia. Liver failure is uncommon after traumatic laceration. Obtaining a blood culture may be useful, but does not assist in making the diagnosis of meningitis. Atelectasis as a result of immobilization and sedation would result in respiratory symptomatology. (**Ref. 5,** pp. 1720, 1230–1231, 1150–1151)

7. (**E**)   Adolescents over the age of 14 or 15 have been shown to possess decision-making capacity and should be included in the discussion of their prognosis. Although her parents may not have discussed the patient's prognosis, her direct question deserves an honest and truthful response. Having her parents available may be optimal, but the discussion should not be delayed unless the patient so requests. (**Ref. 6,** pp. 79–81)

8. (**B**)   Rouleaux formation and the presence of a nucleated red blood cell are shown in Figure 2.1. Rouleaux formation is secondary to excessive plasma globulins and may be seen in multiple myeloma. Bone marrow invasion can cause the early release of nucleated red blood cells into the peripheral blood. Alcoholic liver disease and folate and vitamin B12 deficiency typically result in a macrocytosis, but not in rouleaux formation. The rest of his presentation is classic multiple myeloma. Iron deficiency anemias are usually microcytic hypochronic when chronic. (**Ref. 1,** pp. 1621–1622)

9. (**E**)   At the time of diagnosis, hypercalcemia is present in approximately one third of patients with multiple myeloma. Another

one third develop elevated calcium levels during the course of the disease. Common symptoms include those listed, plus polyuria and polydipsia. Hyperglycemia, hypoglycemia, hyperuricemia, and hypokalemia are not commonly seen in multiple myeloma. (**Ref. 1,** pp. 1621–1622)

10. **(C)** Normal saline and loop diuretics are often the first measures instituted for hypercalcemia with onset of actions in hours. Biphosphates and calcitonin can also be used. Ca^{+2} binding resins exist, but are not easily utilized in hypercalcemia. (**Ref. 1,** p. 2163)

11. **(B)** The peripheral blood smear in disseminated intravascular coagulation (DIC) is characterized by the presence of schistocytes, helmet cells, and decreased platelets. Multiple conditions, including malignancies, vascular malformations and thrombosis, infections, and retained fetus and amniotic fluid, are associated with DIC. Prosthetic valve hemolysis is not associated with thrombocytopenia. (**Ref. 1,** pp. 1807–1808)

12. **(C)** Impaired coagulation, including prolonged prothrombin time, decreased plasma fibrinogen, and thrombocytopenia, are seen in DIC and in chronic liver disease. Anemia, multifactorial in nature, may be seen in patients with alcoholic liver disease. Surreptitious heparin use is typically manifested by an elevated partial thromboplastin time, without other abnormalities of hemostasis. Hemochromatosis doesn't affect these parameters except in end-stage disease. An isolated elevation of the prothrombin time is found in patients with a vitamin K deficiency. (**Ref. 1,** pp. 1446, 1806, 2069–2073)

13. **(B)** Acute promyelocytic leukemia is associated with DIC, especially during induction of chemotherapy. Prevention of infection during chemotherapy-induced nadirs of WBC counts is essential. Therapy for underlying acidosis or infection should always be instituted. DIC associated with malignancy usually requires treatment of the malignancy. Steroids are generally not utilized for acute promyelocytic leukemia and secondary DIC. (**Ref. 1,** pp. 1766–1767, 1770)

14. **(B)** Homosexual or bisexual men, IV drug abusers, Haitians, patients with hemophilia A, and sexual partners of AIDS patients are at high risk to develop AIDS especially if they don't practice secretion precautions. Household contacts of AIDS patients and medical personnel caring for AIDS patients are at very low risk of contracting AIDS, provided they avoid contact with the patient's blood and other body secretions. Deep IM injections of HIV serum have converted health care workers to HIV+ status. (**Ref. 1**, pp. 1569–1570)

15. **(A)** The presence of interstitial infiltrates in a patient with AIDS is most likely due to *P. carinii*. The subacute course is also consistent with cytomegalovirus or other viral pneumonias. The chest x-ray in pneumococcal pneumonia is characterized by focal alveolar infiltrates rather than diffuse interstitial infiltrates. Nonspecific interstitial pneumonitis can have a normal or interstitial infiltrate on CXR. (**Ref. 1**, p. 1607)

16. **(C)** Pentamidine, trimethoprim-sulfamethoxazole, and clindamycin with primaquine have been shown to be effective in the treatment of *P. carinii,* which is seen in Figure 2.3. *P. carinii* organisms are not sensitive to acyclovir. (**Ref. 1**, p. 1594)

17. **(B)** Tuberculous and fungal meningitis typically have mild to moderate elevation of CSF protein, decreased CSF glucose, and an elevated leukocyte count; in contrast to bacterial meningitis, the leukocytes in the CSF are predominantly lymphocytes. Cerebral aneurysms have normal CSF values unless they bleed. Glucose is usually normal in aseptic meningitis. (**Ref. 1**, pp. 824–825, 2296–2297)

18. **(E)** This figure shows a positive India ink preparation for *Cryptococcus neoformans.* CT scans of the brain or technetium brain scans only occasionally reveal focal lesions and would require serologic or culture confirmation of this diagnosis. Blood cultures are positive in 10% of patients. Virtually all patients with cryptococcal meningoencephalitis will have detectable capsular antigen in CSF or serum. (**Ref. 1**, p. 1601)

19. **(A)** Cryptococcal meningoencephalitis requires treatment with IV amphotericin B, either alone or in combination with oral fluconazole. Amphotericin routinely results in renal insufficiency and hypokalemia. Peripheral neuropathy is seen with isoniazid therapy. **(Ref. 1,** p. 1609)

20. **(A)** The patient in Figure 2.5 has a purpuric rash due to meningococcemia. Altered mental status, fever, and a petechial or purpuric rash may be seen. Erythema migrans is the rash of Lyme disease. **(Ref. 1,** pp. 642, 561, 2299)

21. **(D)** Counterimmunoelectrophoresis or latex agglutination of spinal fluid may be useful in rapidly establishing the diagnosis of meningococcal meningitis. The organism may be recovered from cultures of blood, spinal fluid, or petechial scrapings. The presence of meningococcus in the nasopharynx does not, by itself, establish the diagnosis of meningococcal infection. **(Ref. 1,** pp. 641–644)

22. **(B)** Intimate contacts of patients with meningococcal disease should receive prophylaxis with rifampin in the doses given. Sulfonamides may be used for organisms known to be sensitive to sulfonamides. Penicillin VK has not been shown to provide effective prophylaxis for meningococcal disease. Minocycline is an older therapy. **(Ref. 1,** p. 643)

23. **(B)** Acalculous cholecystitis accounts for 5% to 10% of all cases of cholecystitis. Patients are generally elderly and/or diabetic. Multiple predisposing factors include recent unrelated major surgery, trauma, burns, prolonged childbirth, and various infections of the biliary tract. Hepatitis is not known to be a risk factor. **(Ref. 15,** p. 496)

24. **(B)** Subdural hematoma is primarily the result of venous bleeding due to damage to the bridging veins located between the dura and the arachnoid membranes. Acute subdural hematoma is more common after head trauma than epidural hematoma, with incidences of approximately 5% and 1% to 2%, respectively. However, subarachnoid bleeding following head trauma is more common than either subdural or epidural bleeding. Acute posttraumatic subdural hematoma carries a 60% to 80% mortality rate unless early recognition and surgical intervention occur. (**Ref. 12,** p. 352)

25. (**D**) The clinical picture of an elderly patient with longstanding rheumatoid arthritis presenting with splenomegaly and neutropenia is the classic picture of Felty's syndrome. Leukemia could present with splenomegaly and a relatively low white blood cell count, but there is no evidence of blast reaction here. Hydroxychloroquine may have isolated neutropenia as a drug reaction, but that is not usually associated with splenomegaly. Pneumococcal sepsis could occur in this setting, but would typically be found with a left shift in the white blood cell count. There is no evidence of the hemolysis with the normal reticulocyte count. (**Ref. 1,** p. 1652)

26. (**C**) Low serum T-3 is most consistent with either hypothyroidism or the euthyroid sick syndrome. Subacute thyroiditis would most likely cause an elevated T-3. An increased concentration of thyroxin binding globulin would increase the total amount of T-3 present. Grave's disease causes hypothyroidism and also is associated with an elevated T-3. Patients with Hashimoto's, when euthyroid, would have a normal T-3. (**Ref. 1,** p 1941)

27. (**B**) The primary distinction between hypothyroidism and euthyroid sick syndrome is the level of the TSH. It is elevated in hypothyroidism and usually normal or slightly low in the euthyroid sick syndrome. A radionucleide uptake scan would be useful in distinguishing Grave's disease from subacute thyroiditis, but these are not in the differential. Antithyroid antibodies are consistent with autoimmune thyroiditis or Grave's disease. Thyroid globulin levels help to indicate the level of binding protein. A sedimentation rate may be a nonspecific indicator of systemic illness as well as thyroiditis. (**Ref. 1,** p. 1941)

28. (E) Serum urea nitrogen and creatinine would be helpful to sort out the etiology of the hyperkalemia. Similarly serum magnesium and calcium and urinary electrolytes may be useful in sorting underlying problems once the patient is stabilized. However, at the time of presentation with acute hyperkalemia, the most important test is the ECG. The presence of acute changes would indicate that treatment must be initiated immediately. (**Ref. 1,** p. 253)

29. (B) A low fractional excretion of sodium (FeNa) indicates that the kidneys are functioning and aggressively retaining sodium. This scenario is typically seen in the setting of prerenal azotemia. Acute tubular necrosis, glomerular nephritis, and interstitial nephritis affect the kidneys' ability to concentrate; accordingly, there is excess loss of sodium and the fractional excretion of sodium is typically greater than 1.0. It is possible for bladder neck obstruction to lead to a low fractional excretion of sodium. However, the presence of a renal ultrasound, which shows no evidence of obstruction, largely rules out this possibility. (**Ref. 1,** pp. 1270–1271)

30. (A) Involvement of a single lymph node region is classified as Stage I; Stage II disease is involved in two or more lymph node regions in the same side of the diaphragm. Involvement of lymph node regions on both sides of the diaphragm (Stage III) or diffuse involvement of extra lymphatic organ (Stage IV) are associated with a poorer prognosis. Fever, sweats, or weight loss greater than 10% are designated as "B" symptoms, but not itching. (**Ref. 1,** p. 1785)

31. (A) Following staging laparotomy, in patients with stage Ia and IIa disease with supradiaphragmatic involvement only, subtotal nodal irradiation is the treatment of choice. For patients with subdiaphragmatic Stage II disease of the periaortic nodes, chemotherapy is recommended. The therapy is the same for Stage Ib and IIb Hodgkin's disease; however, the relapse rate is higher. Relapse can usually be salvaged with chemotherapy. Combination chemotherapy with involved field radiation remains an alternative treatment for these patients. Stage IIb bulky disease should be managed with combined modality therapy, including chemotherapy and radiotherapy at the sites of both diseases. Stage IIIa patients seem to respond equally well to total lymphoid radiation, combination chemotherapy with radiation, or chemotherapy alone. In Stage IIIb or Stage IV, combination chemotherapy is recommended. (**Ref. 1**, p. 1788)

32. **(B)** Coronary artery bypass grafting has only been shown to prolong life in the setting of left ventricular dysfunction associated with left main or three vessel coronary artery disease. Angina is relieved or significantly reduced in 85% of patients undergoing surgery. There is no evidence that surgery improves survival in patients with angina and one or two vessel disease. (**Ref. 1**, pp. 969–970)

33. **(B)** Competency is a legal determination that can only be made by a court or court officer. Requirements for involuntary commitment vary from state to state but generally require a treatable mental illness in addition to a danger or potential danger to self or others. Patients have the right to refuse treatment, even for life-threatening illnesses. This does not automatically mean they are incompetent or should be committed. It is important to assess the patient's mental condition and understanding of the clinical situation. It may also be beneficial to involve family members in the process. (**Ref. 18**, pp. 82–88)

34. **(A)** Responsibility for the patient's care remains with the physician. The most a utilization reviewer can do is deny payment for services. Even when they do authorize treatment, payment is often not guaranteed until a review of the medical record is complete. The patient should be informed of the situation and of possible alternatives, including fiscal responsibility. Often a decision may be appealed to another level where the treating physician may speak with another doctor. Physicians should act as advocates for their patients in this changing health care climate. (**Ref. 18**, pp. 293–299)

35. **(C)** If there is a history of alcoholism, withdrawal is a likely candidate. Even with alcoholism in the history, CNS infections, neo-

plasms, and injuries ought to be considered. Long-term severe alcohol abuse is associated with hyponatremia, not hypernatremia. (**Ref. 10,** pp. 404–405)

36. **(E)** The benzodiazepines chlordiazepoxide (Librium) and diazepam (Valium) have erratic absorption when given intramuscularly and, thus, that route of administration should be avoided. Oral doses are often sufficient and effective although intravenous administration may sometimes be indicated. Other withdrawal symptoms include delirium, autonomic hyperactivity, and tremulousness which can develop up to a week after withdrawal. While in common practice, padded tongue blades are seldom of use once a seizure has started. Carbamazepine is as effective as a benzodiazepine in treating withdrawal.(**Ref. 10,** pp. 405–406)

37. **(E)** Autonomic hyperactivity includes tachycardia, diaphoresis, hypertension, anxiety, insomnia, and fever. Hypothermia is not a common symptom. Psychomotor status can fluctuate from lethargy to hyperexcitability. (**Ref. 10,** pp. 406–407)

38. **(B)** The best treatment for DTs is prevention. The withdrawing patient should receive a benzodiazepine such as chlordiazepoxide (Librium) 25-50 mg. po q 2–4 hrs. until out of danger. If DTs do occur, higher doses (50–100mgs q 4 hrs) may be required or even intravenous doses. Physical restraints may be risky as patients may become exhausted fighting the restraints. Patients are often dehydrated and this condition should be corrected. High calorie, high carbohydrate diet is important. While a seclusion room may be necessary at times, warm supportive psychotherapy and not physical isolation is essential. (**Ref. 10,** pp. 406–407)

39. **(C)** Poor nutrition or malabsorption problems leading to thiamine deficiency are the common pathophysiological connections between the two disorders. Wernicke's is an acute condition that is readily reversible if treated early. Wernicke's can progress to Korsakoff's syndrome which is a chronic amnestic syndrome with

only a 20% recovery rate. Blackouts are a symptom of acute intoxication and are unrelated to the two conditions. (**Ref. 10**, pp. 407–408)

40. (**C**)   This 65-year-old obese white man was admitted with lower abdominal colicky pain of three-days' duration. The location of the pain in the left lower quadrant and in the suprapubic area should raise a suspicion of an inflammatory lesion. The history of similar attacks of pain in the previous year might lead one to think of diverticulitis. This goes along with increasing constipation and episodes of diarrhea. However, the possibility that this may be due to a cancer should also be kept in mind. Either of these conditions could produce some degree of large bowel obstruction. However, this has not reached the point in this patient to make him vomit. He does have constipation and has not passed any gas. The admitting vital signs revealed an elevated temperature and this should further confirm the suspicion of an inflammatory bowel problem such as diverticulitis or a perforation due to a cancer. Although important, alcohol intake is not required with this presentation.

Patients with diverticular disease do not often bleed. When bleeding occurs, it is usually the massive variety and generally stops spontaneously. On the other hand patients with cancer of the colon might have no obvious bleeding but have steady blood loss. Conditions such as ulcerative colitis, however, are associated with bloody diarrhea. The increased use of laxatives should indicate a progressively narrowing lesion in the large bowel and this could be either an inflammatory stricture or a malignant process. The absence of weight loss reduces the possibility of malignancy. The patient has urinary symptoms including dysuria and frequency. This is not unusual at the time patients first present prostatic symptoms. In a patient with a history suggestive of inflammatory process, one should think of the process extending to the bladder wall. In addition, an enlarged prostate could be responsible for the same symptoms. In this obese individual diagnosis of an abdominal mass is not easy. However, localized tenderness in the left lower quadrant is strongly suggestive of diverticulitis. Once the diverticulitis is localized, the bowel sounds may be normal. Only when there is a free perforation is the abdomen completely silent. (**Ref. 14**, pp. 1016–1020, 1470)

41. (C) A rectal examination is necessary and the stool should be checked for guaiac. In diverticulitis, it might localize the tenderness, and, in the presence of a low-lying cancer, a mass may be felt. The initial workup revealed an elevated white cell count with left shift. This strongly supports the suspicion of an inflammatory process such as diverticulitis. The urine culture showed predominantly fecal organisms and one should suspect an extension of the inflammatory process into the bladder. Stool cultures are of no value in this patient. Plain abdominal series are useful in determining the gas pattern and evidence of bowel obstruction. When there is a free perforation due to diverticulitis, the x-ray film will show free air in the abdomen. A useful procedure at this stage is ultrasonography. In this patient, this revealed a mass. Sometimes the sonogram might reveal the presence of an abscess and indicate the need for early exploration and drainage. (**Ref. 14,** pp. 1166, 1032)

42. (A) The initial management of diverticulitis is by conservative measures. The patient should be on IV fluids and, if necessary, nasogastric suction. Parenteral antibiotics, including gentamicin and either clindaycin or metronidazole, would be useful in controlling local infection. In acute diverticulitis the patient would regurgitate any oral intake, and oral neomycin and erythromycin have no value. Similarly, bulk laxatives are only useful in the conservative management of diverticulitis. A cecostomy is not useful. Most patients are treated conservatively, and if their disease does not resolve or they develop one of the complications, then surgery would be considered. A proximal colostomy alone, even in the presence of perforated diverticulitis, is not as useful as a colostomy combined with drainage of the involved segment or resection. (**Ref. 14,** pp. 1203–1205)

43. (E) In the presence of diverticulitis, sigmoidoscopy is often not helpful. The scope can seldom advance past the sigmoid flexure due to spasm and even then it may only show some pus or mucus trickling down. CT scan and barium enema may further delineate the extent of the diverticulitis and the presence of an abscess. The patient, as noted in the history and management, has passed air or gas along with urine. This should raise a strong suspicion of colovesical fistula. The most useful methods for diagnosing this are a cystogram and cystoscopy. The cystogram presented in Figure 2.6 shows a fistula and appearance of the contrast in a bowel loop. Urethrogram is only indicated when feces or air are leaking through the meatus irrespective of bladder contraction or attempts at micturition. A colonoscopy does not help in pointing to the site of the fistula but only confirms the presence of an inflammatory area, normal or inflamed mucosa, and perhaps a diagnosis of diverticular disease. (**Ref. 14,** pp. 1206–1207)

44. (**A**) The ideal treatment of a patient with colovesical fistula due to diverticular disease is primary resection of the involved segment of colon, repair of the site of fistula in the bladder, and suprapubic drainage. The continuity of the bowel is to be reestablished by primary anastomosis through healthy areas. When there is severe inflammation or an abscess formation at the site of the fistula, one might elect to do a sigmoid resection, proximal colostomy and bladder repair with drainage, and subsequently closing of the colostomy. In the management of colovesical fistula of this nature, hyperalimentation and bladder drainage alone have no value. It might divert the fecal stream, but the feces in the bowel distal to the colostomy will continue to infect the bladder, and further, the fistula will not heal. The patient does not have evidence of hypertrophic prostate, and therefore transurethral prostatectomy has no value in this situation. (**Ref. 14,** pp. 1206–1207)

3

Emergency Department

DIRECTIONS (Questions 1–47): Each of the numbered items or incomplete statements in this chapter is followed by answers or completions of the statement. Select the **ONE** lettered answer or completion that is **BEST** in each case.

---

1. The paramedics bring a 14-year-old female to the ED on a hot day in July. She was standing in line waiting to purchase concert tickets and suddenly passed out. Observers don't remember any unusual movements. On arrival she is awake and oriented although she doesn't remember what happened. Her heart rate is 80 and regular, BP is 100/60, temperature 37°C. Her physical examination is remarkable for her being thin (<5% weight/height). On her EKG the corrected QT interval is 0.35 seconds. The most likely etiology for this event is

   A. a seizure

   B. orthostatic syncope

   C. vasovagal syncope

   D. prolonged QT syndrome

   E. supraventricular tachycardia

2. A 6-week-old is brought to the ED because of persistent nonbilious vomiting beginning five days ago and becoming progressively worse. Despite the vomiting, he is a voracious eater. He is alert and responsive on exam but appears mildly dehydrated. His heart rate is 150, respiratory rate 20, BP 80/40, and he is afebrile. His abdomen is soft and not apparently tender but he is somewhat difficult to examine. His rectal exam is normal and the stool is negative for occult blood. His laboratory studies are as follows:

Na+: 135 mEq/L   WBC: 12,000
K+: 3.6 mEq/L   PMNs: 24%
Cl–: 88 mEq/L   bands: 5%
HCO3–: 32 mEq/L   Hb: 15 gm/dL

The most likely diagnosis is

A. congenital adrenal hyperplasia

B. duodenal atresia

C. gastroesophageal reflux

D. pyloric stenosis

E. intussusception

3. A 10-year-old, limp and with a fever, is brought to the ED. On exam he has point tenderness over the mid-shaft of the left femur. The radiograph of his lower extremity reveals a lucent spot in the area of tenderness. You obtain appropriate lab work and initiate therapy. The most likely causative agent of this disease is

A. *Streptococcus pneumoniae*

B. *Salmonella typhi*

C. *Escherichia coli*

D. *Staphylococcus epidermidis*

E. *Staphylococcus aureus*

4. A 2-year-old is brought to the ED because she is refusing to use her right arm. She had been well until this morning when she and her father were walking down the street. The child fell from the curb into the street. Dad pulled her suddenly back on to the sidewalk. On arriving home, Dad noticed that she was not using her right arm. On exam the child is holding the right arm in a pronated position and cries when the elbow is moved. The appropriate next step is

   A. report the father to Child Protective Services as the description and injury do not make sense

   B. obtain radiographs of the right upper extremity to evaluate for tissue injury

   C. apply pressure over the radial head and supinate the hand and arm

   D. reassure the father that this soft tissue injury will heal without difficulty

   E. apply a splint to the right forearm and suggest application of ice for the first 24 hours

5. A 21-month-old arrives in the ED after being found face down in a neighbor's pool. His mother pulled him from the pool and called 911, who arrived within four minutes. Resuscitation was begun including intubation and chest compressions. He was transported to your hospital and arrived pulseless and not breathing. Cardiac activity, including maintaining a blood pressure, returns 18 minutes after he was found. The pathophysiologic mechanism that will most likely lead to his death is

   A. pulmonary aspiration of water

   B. hypoxic-ischemic injury to the myocardium

   C. hypoxic-ischemic injury to the brain

   D. hyperglycemia which potentiates neuronal injury

   E. hyponatremia secondary to water ingestion

6. A 26-month-old arrives in the ED after a generalized, tonic-clonic seizure. She appeared well until she developed a fever of 104°F. Shortly after the fever was noted, she was noted to have jerking movements of her arms and legs. Her eyes rolled back. The event lasted approximately two minutes. During her transport to the hospital she was sleepy. On arrival she is alert and recognizes her mother. She has a left otitis media. The remainder of her examination by an experienced clinician is normal. Her mother tells you that the child's father had seizures as a young child but "grew out of them." The appropriate next step is

   A. perform a lumbar puncture

   B. order an electroencephalogram

   C. perform a tympanocentesis

   D. reassure the family and prescribe amoxacillin

   E. request a neurology consult

7. A 36-year-old man presents to the ED with right-sided low back and leg pain the day after lifting a heavy object at work. He has a history of a "slipped disk" five years prior which was treated with rest and narcotic pain medication. All of the following associations on physical examination of this patient could be true **EXCEPT**

   A. L4 root irritation and decreased or absent knee jerk reflex

   B. radicular pain with ipsilateral and crossed straight leg raise and the presence of a herniated disk

   C. L5 root irritation and difficulty with heel walking

   D. S1 root irritation and quadriceps muscle dysfunction

   E. S1 root irritation and decreased ankle jerk reflex

8. A 72-year-old presents to the ED complaining of vomiting bright red blood on three occasions over approximately six hours. He also complains of dizziness, but denies abdominal pain. He has been generally healthy. The most likely source of this patient's gastrointestinal bleeding is

   A. esophageal varices

   B. gastric ulcer

   C. esophagitis

   D. gastritis

   E. Mallory-Weiss syndrome

9. Which of the following statements about a patient who presents with hemodynamically significant lower gastrointestinal tract hemorrhage is **FALSE**?

   A. The most common cause of hemorrhage varies with age

   B. The most likely cause of hemorrhage in a patient over 60 years old is diverticulosis

   C. Carcinoma is a likely cause of hemorrhage

   D. Hemorrhage caused by Meckel's diverticulum may occur at any age, but is more common in children

   E. Intussusception is a likely cause of hemorrhage in a child aged 3 months to 3 years

10. A 43-year-old obese mother of four presents to the ED at 2 a.m. complaining of severe nausea and right upper quadrant abdominal pain since 10 p.m. You suspect cholelithiasis or one of its complications to be the source of her discomfort. Concerning her ED workup, which of the following statements is true?

    A. Plain abdominal radiography is likely to show the presence of gallstones in 50% of cases

    B. Normal alkaline phosphatase, bilirubin, and serum aminotransferases exclude the diagnosis of cholecystitis

    C. Nuclear scintigraphy with 99m-technitium-labeled iminodiacetic acid has a higher positive predictive value for cholecystitis than ultrasound imaging.

    D. Oral cholecystography has a significantly higher sensitivity for identifying cholelithiasis than an ultrasound showing a well visualized gall bladder

    E. The polymorphonucleocyte count is uniformly elevated in patients with cholecystitis

Case Cluster (Questions 11–14):

11. A 53-year-old woman presents to the ED with colicky abdominal pain and vomiting for two days, and no bowel movement or flatus for one day. She is tachycardiac and looks ill. Plain radiography of the abdomen reveals multiple distended loops of small bowel with gas/fluid levels in a stair step pattern, and no gas in the colon. Which of the following is her most likely diagnosis?

    A. Colonic obstruction

    B. Perforated duodenal ulcer

    C. Gastroenteritis

D. Small bowel obstruction

E. Appendicitis

12. Which of the following combinations of laboratory findings is most likely in this patient?

   A. K+: 4.3; Cl–: 102; Serum Bicarb: 24; Urine Specific Gravity: 1.020

   B. K+: 3.2; Cl–: 89; Serum Bicarb: 34; Urine Specific Gravity: 1.040

   C. K+: 5.6; Cl–: 109; Serum Bicarb: 15; Urine Specific Gravity: 1.040

   D. K+: 5.6; Cl–: 109; Serum Bicarb: 34; Urine Specific Gravity: 1.040

   E. K+: 3.2; Cl–: 89; Serum Bicarb: 15; Urine Specific Gravity: 1.020

13. Which of the following is the **INCORRECT** statement regarding the management and expected outcome of this patient?

   A. Initial management should consist of nasogastric decompression and fluid and electrolyte replacement

   B. The patient is likely to require surgical intervention

   C. Once resolved, this patient is likely to suffer recurrence

   D. Surgical intervention may be avoided if resolution is evident with conservative management in 24 to 48 hours

   E. Persistent pain, fever, lactic acidosis, and leukocytosis suggest the need for urgent surgical intervention

14. The most likely etiology for this patient's condition is

    A. hernia

    B. tumor

    C. postoperative adhesions

    D. metabolic derangement

    E. infection

Case Cluster (Questions 15–17):

15. A 19-year-old man is being transported to the ED following a shallow water diving accident. The accident was witnessed by a lifeguard who immediately pulled him from the water and began mouth to mask breathing. The patient has been secured on a backboard with his cervical spine immobilized. Your most immediate concern when this patient arrives must be

    A. checking for pulse rate and blood pressure

    B. checking for clear and equal breath sounds

    C. assessing and securing a patent airway

    D. calculating a Glasgow coma score for this patient

    E. obtaining a cervical spine x-ray

16. On arrival in the ED the patient undergoes successful orotracheal intubation with appropriate consideration for protection of the cervical spine. He is found to have a pulse rate of 58, and a blood pressure of 76/42. The patient is noted to be flaccid below the clavicles with no spontaneous respiration. Priapism is present. Which of the following statements about this patient is true?

    A. This patient will require intravenous dopamine to restore normotension

B. The diagnosis of spinal shock can be immediately assumed in any patient with an appropriate mechanism of injury and hypotension

C. This patient is likely to be hyperreflexic on examination of the deep tendon reflexes

D. Failure of this patient's blood pressure to normalize with Trendelenburg position and crystalloid infusion should prompt a search for missed injuries

E. This patient may exhibit hyperthermia due to loss of autonomic temperature control mechanisms

17. A 3-view cervical spine series shows a posterior subluxation of C2 on C3. Correct statements regarding the further care of this spinal cord injured patient in the ED include all of the following **EXCEPT**

A. pressure necrosis of denervated skin may occur within one hour if the patient remains on an unpadded spinal immobilization board

B. high dose methylprednisolone may improve functional outcome

C. it is not appropriate to remove spine immobilization until complete radiologic evaluation and a definitive assessment of the stability of the injury has been made

D. arrangements for transfer of this patient to a spinal cord injury center should be made

E. further radiologic evaluation should include lateral cervical spine x-rays with the neck in flexion and extension

18. Concerning hemorrhagic shock, which of the following is the most correct match of percent blood volume loss and expected signs and symptoms?

   A. 10%: clear sensorium, normal to mildly tachycardiac heart rate, normotensive, normal capillary refill

   B. 15%: decreased level of consciousness, tachycardiac, normotensive with widened pulse pressure, visible pallor

   C. 20%: decreased level of consciousness, tachycardiac; no palpable pulses, visible pallor

   D. 30%: clear sensorium, tachycardiac, normotensive with widened pulse pressure, normal capillary refill

   E. 40%: anxious, tachycardiac, normotensive with widened pulse pressure, delayed capillary refill

19. A child presents to the ED with pain, deformity, and swelling of the elbow following a fall from a tree branch. Which of the following is **NOT** true of pediatric fractures?

   A. Torus and greenstick fractures are incomplete fractures found more commonly in children due to the increased pliability of the bones in childhood

   B. The epiphyseal growth plate in children is subject to injury from compressive or shearing forces

   C. Dislocations and subluxations are rare in childhood relative to their frequency in adults

   D. The incidence of open fractures is higher in children due to a weaker and less resilient periosteum

   E. The incidence of non-union in childhood is rare due to the osteogenic capacity of the periosteum in children

20. Which of the following is an **INCORRECT** association between an orthopedic injury and a physical finding related to an associated nerve injury?

    A. Supracondylar humerus fracture : inability to oppose the thumb

    B. Proximal humerus fracture : inability to extend the wrist

    C. Lateral tibial plateau fracture : loss of sensation to the lateral calf

    D. Anterior shoulder dislocation : inability to abduct the shoulder

    E. Acromio-clavicular joint dissociation : inability to extend the wrist

21. A 19-year-old presents to the ED with the complaint of testicular pain. The pain began in the left lower abdomen while the patient was playing soccer, and has subsequently radiated to the left testicle. The pain began approximately four hours prior to presentation. The patient denies trauma to the testicles, and he denies being sexually active. The patient also tells you that he had similar pain several months ago, but that it subsided spontaneously. The most correct statement regarding this patient's diagnosis is

    A. his testicular salvage rate is less than 50% even if the appropriate management is instituted immediately

    B. the presence of pain in the same testicle previously is uncommon for this diagnosis

    C. the presence of Prehn's sign would be diagnostic for epididymitis in this patient

    D. the patient should have simultaneous Doppler flow ultrasound of the testicle or testicular scintigraphic scan and urologic consultation immediately

    E. the patient can be safely discharged on antibiotics and pain medication for follow-up with a urologist tomorrow

22. A 66-year-old man presents to the ED with the complaint of abdominal pain which began suddenly about two hours prior to presentation. He states this pain is constant and intense, and radiates to the right flank and groin. The patient denies any respiratory, gastrointestinal, or urologic symptoms. He denies any recent abdominal pain before tonight. The patient is a smoker and has had poorly controlled hypertension for many years. He has had an MI three years prior. Examination reveals the patient to be very uncomfortable and diaphoretic. His vital signs include a blood pressure of 175/110 and a pulse rate of 106. He is afebrile. Palpation of masses in the abdomen is difficult due to obesity, but the abdomen is generally tender without guarding. The diagnosis which best fits this case is

A. acute cholecystitis

B. ureterolithiasis

C. abdominal aortic aneurysm

D. pancreatitis

E. perforated peptic ulcer

Case Cluster (Questions 23–29):

23. A 29-year-old man is brought to the ED after a motorcycle crash. He was not wearing a helmet, and has suffered apparent head, face, and extremity injury. He presents in appropriate spine immobilization. The prehospital care provider reports the patient to have a pulse of 124 palpable at the femoral arteries. He is nonverbal and nonpurposefully combative. He has a scalp laceration, an obviously fractured mandible and a grossly abnormal appearing right hip and femur. The most important first step in the management of this case is

A. check distal pulses in the right lower extremity

B. obtain peripheral intravenous access

C. obtain a blood pressure via sphygmomanometer

D. check the oro-pharynx for foreign bodies

E. auscultate the lungs

24. All of the following findings would suggest the need for immediate airway control via tracheal intubation in this patient **EXCEPT**

   A. the patient's altered mental status and combative state

   B. the presence of blood and fractured teeth in the oropharynx

   C. the lack of breath sounds in the right chest on auscultation

   D. upper airway noise on breathing which improves with the jaw-thrust maneuver

   E. vomiting

25. The patient is successfully intubated by the orotracheal route. A lack of breath sounds is indeed present on the right side, along with palpable crepitus. The patient has a brief improvement in blood pressure to 110/50. Shortly thereafter, the patient becomes difficult to ventilate and blood pressure is no longer able to be auscultated. You suspect tension pneumothorax. All of the following are true of tension pneumothorax **EXCEPT**

   A. may develop during mechanical ventilation

   B. results when intrapleural and atmospheric pressures equalize

   C. causes hypotension via increasing intrathoracic pressure and concomitantly decreasing venous return to the heart

   D. is treated by immediate needle or tube thoracostomy

   E. left unrecognized, may result in a pulseless electrical cardiac rhythm

26. Following tube thoracostomy, the patient's blood pressure remains 80/40. He remains tachycardiac and combative. Of the following potential causes for this patient's continued tachycardia and altered mental status, which must be considered and managed next?

   A. Intracranial injury

   B. Spinal shock

   C. Drug or alcohol intoxication

   D. Hypovolemia due to hemorrhage

   E. Cardiac contusion

27. The most correct initial management of hypotension in this patient would be

   A. crystalloid infusion up to two liters, then switch to blood if hypotension and tachycardia persist

   B. withhold all fluid management until a source of hemorrhage is determined

   C. vasopressor infusion to achieve normotension

   D. hypertonic crystalloid and dextran infusion until normotensive and non-tachycardiac

   E. colloid infusion until normotensive and non-tachycardiac

28. A 26-year-old white female presents to the ED in near coma. Her blood sugar is determined to be 420 mg per deciliter. Other laboratory results reveal a sodium of 131, potassium 3.4, bicarbonate 10, chloride 99. Urine ketones are positive. Which of the following statements is true?

   A. C-peptide is undetectable

   B. The ketones detected in the urine are predominately beta hydroxy butyrate

C. Obesity likely plays a role by confirming a high degree of insulin resistance

D. She is likely to have a strong family history of diabetes mellitus

E. After she is stabilized, she may do well on an oral hypoglycemic agent

29. All of the following would be appropriate in the initial management of this woman **EXCEPT**

A. intravenous (IV) infusion of isotonic fluids

B. IV sodium bicarbonate to raise the pH to 7.40

C. subcutaneous, IM, or IV infusion of insulin

D. cautious potassium replacement

E. measurement of serum phosphate and magnesium

30. A 65-year-old woman is brought into the ED with a low blood pressure and steady pulse that seems intermittent. She has a paradoxic pulse of 18 mm Hg. You are concerned that she may have

A. critical aortic stenosis

B. acute myocardial infarction

C. cardiac tamponade

D. pulmonary embolism

E. atrial fibrillation with a rapid ventricular response

31. A 35-year-old white woman presents to the ED with an episode of syncope lasting approximately 15 minutes. She denies prodomal symptoms. History reveals that this is her third episode. Which of the following statements concerning syncope in this patient is most likely true?

  A. 24-hour ambulatory ECG monitoring and intracardiac electrophysiologic studies would be the most useful diagnostic tests

  B. The likelihood that the etiology of this syncope will be determined is less than 50%

  C. Cardiac arrhythmias are the most common cause of syncope in patients who present in this fashion

  D. The one-year incidence of sudden death in patients with unexplained recurrent syncope is up to 25%

  E. A complete workup will also include an electroencephalogram (EEG), tilt table testing, and electrophysiologic testing of the heart

32. A 27-year-old black basketball player passes out on the court during an intense practice. He recovers and is referred for evaluation. Examination reveals a coarse mid-systolic murmur, which increases in duration and intensity on moving from a supine position to a standing position. The likely diagnosis is

  A. hypertrophic obstructive cardiomyopathy

  B. aortic stenosis

  C. mitro regurgitation

  D. atrial septal defect

  E. aortic regurgitation

33. A 58-year-old black man is brought to the ED following a generalized tonic-clonic seizure. He has no previous history of seizure. The most likely etiology is

   A. brain tumor

   B. cerebral vascular disease

   C. alcoholism

   D. trauma

   E. brain abscess

Case Cluster (Questions 34–36):

34. A 45-year-old man with a 20-year history of severe chronic alcohol abuse presents to the ED with chief complaints of shortness of breath and epigastric abdominal pain of 24-hour duration. Physical examination reveals a blood pressure of 90/60, a respiratory rate of 22 breaths per minute that appear unusually deep, and minimal epigastric tenderness to palpation. Pertinent laboratory studies revealed: PaO_2 = 86; $PaCO_2$ = 30; pH = 7.32; sodium = 140; potassium = 4.5; chloride = 105; HCO_3 = 15. The arterial blood gases and serum electrolyte results are consistent with which of the following acid base disorders?

   A. Acute respiratory alkalosis

   B. Metabolic acidosis, normal anion gap

   C. Chronic respiratory alkalosis with metabolic compensation

   D. Metabolic acidosis, increased anion gap

   E. None of the above

35. The acid base disorder in this patient may commonly result from

    A. diarrhea, renal tubular acidosis, a previous ureterosigmoidostomy surgical procedure, or primary hyperparathyroidism

    B. anxiety, excessive mechanical ventilation, acute asthma, or rapid ascent in altitude

    C. hepatic cirrhosis, pregnancy, or chronic cerebral disease (brain tumor, stroke, encephalitis, etc.)

    D. uncontrolled diabetes mellitus, acute and chronic alcoholism, severe acute circulatory failure, poisoning and drug toxicity, or renal failure

    E. none of the above

36. Helpful diagnostic studies to evaluate the acid base disorder in this patient would include

    A. urine pH, stool electrolytes, serum calcium

    B. serum levels of glucose, urea nitrogen, ketones, as well as a serum drug screen

    C. serum ammonia and a computerized axial tomography (CAT) scan of the head

    D. serum pregnancy test

    E. none of the above

37. A 23-year-old is brought to the ED by his family because they are concerned that he may be using drugs. In recent weeks, he has withdrawn from his friends and appears more anxious and tense. He is noncommittal regarding any drug use. His family has found what you later identify as amphetamines in his room. You would expect to observe the following symptoms on physical examination **EXCEPT**

   A. pupillary constriction

   B. tachycardia or bradycardia

   C. nausea or vomiting

   D. psychomotor agitation or retardation

   E. confusion

Case Cluster (Questions 38–42):

38. A 2-year-old is brought to the ED in the middle of the night because of difficulty breathing. On entering the room, it is apparent to you that she has stridor. In evaluating the sense of urgency about this child's airway obstruction, the most concerning historical information would be

   A. she has had a cold for several days and had difficulty sleeping last evening because of her cough

   B. the stridor seems to be worse when she cries

   C. she was a premature infant who required reintubation several times in the neonatal period

   D. her temperature has been 39°C for the last 36 hours

   E. she has been drooling since she woke up in distress and now refuses to lie down

39. You proceed to the physical examination. In light of the presenting problem the **LEAST** important element of the physical exam is

    A. determination of the respiratory rate

    B. determination of the heart rate

    C. inspection of the chest

    D. auscultation of the breath sounds

    E. observation for evidence of cyanosis

40. The child continues to exhibit inspiratory and expiratory stridor, especially when agitated. She has minimal inspiratory stridor when calm in her mother's arms. She is not drooling. Her heart rate is 120, respiratory rate is 24 and temperature is 38.2°C. The remainder of her exam is unremarkable. By history, you are convinced that this is not a foreign body ingestion. You begin to order diagnostic studies. The most appropriate tests to order are

    A. blood gases and inspiratory and expiratory chest radiographs

    B. blood gases and a lateral neck radiograph

    C. oxygen saturation by pulse oximetry, and inspiratory and expiratory chest radiographs

    D. oxygen saturation by pulse oximetry and a lateral neck radiograph

    E. oxygen saturation by pulse oximetry, chest radiograph, and lateral neck radiograph

41. The child has evidence of adequate oxygenation and the radiographs are read as normal. You make the appropriate diagnosis. The most likely etiology for this disease is

    A. hemophilus influenzae, type B

    B. *Staphylococcus aureus*

    C. parainfluenza virus

    D. adenovirus

    E. influenza virus

42. Because of the respiratory distress you decide to admit the child to the hospital for further management of her disease. The appropriate treatment for this disorder is

    A. humidified air, antipyretics, antibiotics, and careful observation

    B. humidified air, antipyretics, bronchodilators, and careful observation

    C. humidified air, endotracheal intubation, antipyretics, and careful observation

    D. humidified air, steroids, antibiotics, and careful observation

    E. humidified air, antipyretics, and careful observation

Case Cluster (Questions 43–47):

43. You have been caring for an 11-year-old girl with asthma. She was diagnosed at 5 years of age and has had some difficulty in controlling her disease. During the first three years of her disease she was hospitalized one to two times/year for acute exacerbations. She never required admission to an ICU. For the next two years she did reasonably well with only two visits to an ED and no hospitalizations. Over the last year she has had increasing problems and has been hospitalized four times. Her routine regimen at home is two puffs of albuterol, administered by metered-dose inhaler three times each day. Chromolyn sodium was begun last summer when she experienced increasing problems with excercise. You have encouraged the family to attend educational sessions and have provided a flow meter for use at home as well as a personalized crisis management plan. The child's mother calls you because the child has had increasing respiratory symptoms over the last two days. She has been coughing at night and has required several additional doses of albuterol for dyspnea. They have not routinely increased the albuterol and are uncertain what her peak flow is. The next appropriate step is

A. bring the child to the office immediately for evaluation of her wheezing

B. begin prednisone orally and increase the frequency of albuterol administration to every four hours

C. give an additional albuterol now and call back in two hours unless the child has improved

D. measure her peak flow and follow the directions based on the crisis management plan

E. increase the albuterol to three puffs now and adjust the frequency if she is still wheezing tonight

44. Several days later (after not hearing back from your last encounter) you meet the child in the ED. She is alert, audibly wheezing, and has suprasternal and intercostal retractions. Her oxygen saturation is 93% in room air. Her heart rate is 130, respiratory rate is 22/min and BP is 110/80. She is afebrile. On auscultation she has inspiratory and expiratory polyphonic wheezes in all lung fields. The appropriate next step is

A. administer oxygen and subcutaneous epinephrine

B. administer oxygen and provide albuterol by metered-dose inhaler, 2 puffs every 20 minutes as needed

C. provide albuterol by metered dose inhaler, 2 puffs every 20 minutes as needed

D. provide albuterol (0.15mg/kg) by nebulizer every 20 minutes up to one hour

E. administer oxygen and provide albuterol (0.15mg/kg) by nebulizer every 20 minutes up to one hour

45. After appropriate treatment she continues to wheeze. The finding which would suggest a poor response to therapy and result in hospitalization is

A. a peak expiratory flow rate of 70% of predicted

B. she speaks in single words at best

C. persistent expiratory wheezing

D. a pCO_2 of 30 mm Hg

E. a respiratory rate of 20 breaths per minute

46. The child is admitted to the hospital with a diagnosis of status asthmaticus. You begin appropriate therapy including oral prednisone and albuterol. During administration of albuterol the nurses note a fall in oxygen saturation. The most likely etiology for the desaturation is

    A. decrease in cardiac output and pulmonary blood flow

    B. worsening of the ventilation-perfusion mismatch

    C. increase in cardiac output in the presence of bronchospasm

    D. transient decrease in delivered oxygen concentration during an aerosol

    E. increase in atelectasis during administration of a beta adrenergic agent

47. The child arrives in your office for follow-up after her hospital discharge for status asthmaticus. She has done relatively well at home although she is not keeping a record of her peak flow measurements. You are concerned that she has been poorly controlled and will require increased hospitalization. The information which you elicit to assess the functional impact includes all of the following **EXCEPT**

    A. school attendance and performance

    B. changes in her social situation including her home environment

    C. need for intensive care unit admission in the past

    D. presence of pets and smoking in the home

    E. frequency of use of metered dose inhaler

Emergency Department

Answers and Discussion

1. **(C)** Syncope is the consequence of decreased blood flow to the brain resulting in a brief loss of consciousness. The most frequent etiology is vasovagal syncope which results from vasovagal stimulation precipitated by fear, pain, excitement, or periods of prolonged standing. Orthostatic syncope may occur due to hypovolemia when the child experiences changes in position. Although victims of syncope may have brief tonic contractions of the face, trunk, and extremities, true tonic-clonic seizure activity is usually absent. Prolonged QT syndrome is characterized by sudden loss of consciousness during exercise or a stressful experience. The QT interval, corrected for heart rate, is 0.48 seconds or more to confirm this diagnosis. (**Ref. 5,** pp. 1700–1701)

2. **(D)** Pyloric stenosis presents with nonbilious vomiting that may or may not be projectile. The onset of the symptoms is most often after 3 weeks of life but may appear as late as 5 months of age. The progressive loss of fluid, hydrogen ion, and chloride lead to a hypochloremic metabolic alkalosis. The serum potassium is usually maintained. Although the diagnosis can be made by palpating an olive-sized mass above and to the right of the umbilical area, agitation may make it difficult to detect. Duodenal atresia presents in the neonatal period and typically includes bilious vomiting. Intussusception results from the telescoping of one portion of the intestine into a segment just caudad to it. It presents with sudden

onset of severe colicky pain recurring at frequent intervals. Vomiting occurs in most cases and becomes bilious later in the course of the disease. Gastroesophageal reflux appears most often in the first week of life and results in nonbilious vomiting. Abnormalities in electrolytes are unusual. (**Ref. 5,** pp. 1055–1073)

3. **(E)** *Staphylococcus aureus* is the most common etiologic agent causing osteomyelitis, accounting for 40% to 80% of all cases. Less common pathogens include *Streptococcus pneumoniae, Streptococcus pyogenes,* and gram negative bacilli such as *Salmonella typhi. Escherichia coli* is an uncommon pathogen in osteomyelitis. *Staphylococcus epidermidis* is an unusual causative agent, although it has been reported in neonates. (**Ref. 5,** pp. 724–725)

4. **(C)** Subluxation of the radial head occurs when longitudinal traction is applied to the arm while the elbow is extended. The annular ligament, which provides stability between the radius and ulna and passes around the proximal radius just below the radial head, slides, becoming partially trapped in the radiohumeral joint. Children who sublux the radial head present with their hand held pronated and refusing to move their hand and elbow. Appropriate treatment is gentle supination of the hand and forearm while applying pressure over the radial head. Often, obtaining radiographs results in reduction of the subluxed radial head, but is not necessary if the correct diagnosis is made. (**Ref. 5,** pp. 1951–1952)

5. **(C)** Drowning is the leading cause of death for children under the age of 5 years and the fourth leading cause of death for children of all ages. After submersion, the small amounts of water ingested during the panic phase result in laryngospasm. Loss of consciousness ultimately occurs due to hypoxemia which results in cardiovascular collapse after three to four minutes. Pathophysiologic injuries to multiple organs are due to hypoxemia but the majority of deaths occur due to hypoxia and ischemia of the brain. While aspiration is found in approximately 90% of victims, it is not the causative agent of death. (**Ref. 6,** pp. 857–861)

6. **(D)** Two to four percent of children under the age of 6 years will experience a febrile seizure. The diagnosis of a febrile seizure requires elimination of other possible causes and can be accomplished without testing by experienced clinicians through a thorough history and physical exam. An EEG adds little value to the management of children with febrile seizures. Unless the seizure is complex, consultation with a neurologist is not needed. Reassurance of the family is important as febrile seizures recur in 25% to 50% of children. The most important prognostic factor for recurrence is the age at initial seizure, with children under one year at the time of presentation having the highest recurrence rate. (**Ref. 6**, pp. 1965–1966)

7. **(D)** Quadriceps muscle weakness is an L4 sign, as is decreased knee jerk reflex. L5 root irritation is evidenced by a decreased biceps femoris reflex, decreased strength in the foot dorsiflexors and, occasionally, great toe pain. S1 irritation may result in weakened foot plantar flexion and decreased ankle jerk reflex. The presence of radicular pain with both ipsilateral and crossed straight leg raise in a young man is highly suspicious for the presence of a herniated intravertebral disk in the lumbosacral region. (**Ref. 15**, p. 1284)

8. **(B)** The most common cause of upper gastrointestinal tract bleeding is peptic ulcer disease. Bleeding from a peptic ulcer is more common in patients over the age of 50, is frequently painless, and may be the initial manifestation of the ulcer in 17% to 42% of cases. Esophageal varices, gastritis with mucosal erosion, and Mallory-Weiss syndrome are also important causes of upper gastrointestinal tract bleeding. Esophagitis uncommonly causes hemorrhage. (**Ref. 12**, pp. 1515–1516)

9. **(C)** While colon carcinoma is a common cause of occult lower gastrointestinal tract (LGI) bleeding, it is unlikely to cause hemodynamically significant bleeding. The cause of significant LGI bleeding varies with age. Diverticulosis is the most common cause of LGI hemorrhage over the age of 60, although angiodysplasia of

the colon rivals diverticulosis for this dubious honor. Meckel's diverticulum may cause LGI bleeding at any age, and is the most common cause in children, with intussusception a close second. (**Ref. 12,** pp. 1517–1518)

10. **(C)** Failure to visualize the gallbladder when the hepatic and common ducts are seen on nuclear scintigraphy one hour following oral radiolabled iminodiacetic acid is diagnostic of cystic duct obstruction. In the appropriate clinical setting, this is also diagnostic for cholecystitis. Conversely, ultrasound showing cholelithiasis, wall thickening, and pericholic edema has a positive predictive value of greater than 90%, but is not diagnostic. When the gallbladder can be appropriately visualized, ultrasonography is as sensitive as oral cholecystogram in identifying the presence of gallstones. Only 10% of gallstones are visualized on plain radiography, and laboratory values are more likely to be normal than abnormal in both cholelithiasis and cholecystitis. (**Ref. 12,** p. 1617)

11. **(D)** This patient exhibits the cardinal symptoms and classic radiologic findings of small bowel obstruction. (**Ref. 12,** pp. 1633–1637)

12. **(B)** The patient is expected to be dehydrated due to vomiting, and therefore have a concentrated urine. Vomiting causes a loss of hydrogen and chloride from the stomach, and results in a metabolic alkalosis. The kidney's attempt to correct the metabolic alkalosis via conserving hydrogen ions results in a compensatory loss of potassium from the kidneys. The net effect, therefore, is a hypokalemic, hypochloremic metabolic alkalosis. (**Ref. 12,** pp. 2128, 2129)

13. **(C)** Initial management of small bowel obstruction may be conservative, with nasogastric decompression and fluid and electrolyte replacement, so long as the patient does not show evidence of strangulation. Signs of strangulation of the bowel include persistent pain after decompression, fever, lactic acidosis, and leuko-

cytosis. Despite conservative management, most patients will go on to require surgical intervention. However, once resolved by whatever means, patients have less than a 15% chance of reobstruction. (**Ref. 12,** pp. 1633–1637; **Ref. 14,** pp. 1029–1031)

14. **(C)** Postoperative adhesions are the most frequent cause of small bowel obstruction (64%–79%). Hernias and tumors are responsible for 15% to 25% and 10% to 15% of small bowel obstructions, respectively. Metabolic derangement and infection may be caused by small bowel obstruction due to vomiting and fluid sequestration or bowel ischemia and perforation. (**Ref. 12,** p. 1633; **Ref. 14,** pp. 1029–1031)

15. **(C)** This patient has likely suffered a cervical spine injury and may have aspirated water. The need for mouth to mask breathing at the scene suggests that the patient is not breathing on his own. Assessment and intervention for airway, breathing, and circulation defines the initial management of any seriously ill or injured patient. These basic tenets of patient management are used independent of the skill of the rescuer, and have become ubiquitous in both pediatric and adult, and basic to advanced life support training. For this patient, more advanced techniques such as endotracheal intubation and mechanical ventilation may take the place of mouth to mask breathing when the patient arrives in the ED, but the principles of airway, breathing, and circulation remain the same. (**Ref. 12,** p. 112)

16. **(D)** The presence of apnea, hypotension, relative bradycardia, flaccidity, priapism, and an appropriate mechanism of injury should suggest a high cervical spine injury with associated spinal shock. Spinal shock, however, is a diagnosis of exclusion. It should only be considered after the presence of hemorrhagic shock, tension pneumothorax, or pericardial tamponade have been ruled out. Hypotension secondary to spinal shock will usually respond to Trendelenburg position and crystalloid infusion. The lack of response to these resuscitative measures should trigger the consideration that a more serious injury has been missed. Only rarely, and after a careful search for missed injuries, is dopamine used to

support the blood pressure in spinal shock. The patient would also be expected to exhibit hyporreflexia, hypothermia, and both bladder and bowel atonia. (**Ref. 12,** p. 410)

17. **(E)** Flexion and extension cervical spine x-rays should not be performed if the original cervical spine series suggests abnormality, or if the patient has an impaired mental status due to trauma or intoxication. Spine injured patients should remain in spinal precautions until the extent of the injury is delineated. However, the backboard should be padded to avoid pressure necrosis if the workup or transport of the patient will be extended. High dose methyl-prednisolone has been shown to improve motor and sensory outcomes when instituted within eight hours of the time of injury. Patients with a significant spinal cord injury should be transferred to a trauma center or spinal cord injury center for definitive care. (**Ref. 15,** p. 1152; **Ref. 12,** p. 410)

18. **(A)** Total blood volume in liters can be approximated as 7% of the body weight in kilograms. Thus, a 70 kg person would have a total blood volume of about 5 liters. A patient with a blood loss up to 15% of the total blood volume (750 ml) may be asymptomatic or experience mild tachycardia. This is classified as Class I shock. Class II shock is defined as a blood loss of 15% to 30% of the total blood volume (750 ml to 1500 ml), and is characterized by tachycardia, increased pulse pressure with normotension, anxiety, and a mild delay in capillary refill. Class III shock (30%–40% or 1.5 L–2 L TBV loss) is characterized by tachycardia, hypotension, confusion, and delayed capillary refill. Finally, patients in Class IV shock (>40% or >2 L TBV loss) exhibit a decreased level of consciousness, pallor, cool and diaphoretic skin, tachycardia, and hypotension. (**Ref. 12,** p. 269)

19. **(D)** The skeleton of the child has different properties than that of an adult, therefore the pattern of skeletal injuries is different in children. In childhood, bone is considerably more malleable, therefore incomplete fractures may occur. The torus fracture refers to the similarity between the distally bulged appearance of an axially loaded long bone and the toric-type architectural column. A

greenstick fracture describes a fracture through the stretched side of a levered long bone. Epiphyseal growth plate injuries account for 18% of orthopedic injuries in children, while dislocation and subluxations account for 3%. The periosteum in children has osteogenic capacity, and is thicker, stronger, and more adherent to the bone. Thus childhood fractures are less likely to be open, and heal with a low likelihood of nonunion. (**Ref. 13**, p. 113; **Ref. 12**, pp. 524–526)

20. **(E)** The acromio-clavicular joint is physically distant from the brachial plexus, and its dissociation is not associated with radial nerve dysfunction. Humerus fractures most commonly injure the radial nerve, resulting in loss of function of the muscles in the posterior compartment of the forearm and sensation to the dorsum of the hand. A supracondylar fracture of the humerus may impinge upon the median nerve, resulting in inability to perform median nerve functions such as oppose the thumb, flex the wrist and fingers, or have sensation to the volar thumb, index and long fingers. An anterior shoulder dislocation can damage the axillary nerve causing an inability to abduct the shoulder. A lateral tibial plateau fracture may injure the common peroneal nerve resulting in loss of sensation to the lateral calf. (**Ref. 12**, p. 530)

21. **(D)** The patient is likely experiencing a left testicular torsion given the sudden onset of testicular pain during activity and the presence of a similar pain in the past. Testicular torsion is most common in puberty, although the age may range from five months to 40 years. If torsion is relieved within six hours of onset of pain, the salvage rate is 80% to 100%. Forty-one percent of patients will relate a similar pain in the past which resolved spontaneously. The differential diagnosis of testicular torsion includes epididymitis, epididymo-orchitis, testicular tumor, and torsion of the testicular appendage. Differentiation from these disorders may be difficult as there are no physical findings which are pathognomonic. Pain relief with elevation of the testicle, Prehn's sign, has been falsely considered to be specific for epididymitis. When suspected, testicular torsion must be diagnosed by a method to determine testicular blood flow and surgically corrected as soon as possible. (**Ref. 12**, pp. 1895–1896)

22. **(C)** The presence of sudden onset, constant and intense abdominal pain in a male greater than 60 years of age who is a hypertensive smoker with a history of MI should alert the physician to the possible presence of a ruptured abdominal aortic aneurysm. (**Ref. 12,** p. 1377)

23. **(D)** Assessment and intervention for airway, breathing, and circulation defines the initial management of any seriously ill or injured patient. These basic tenets of patient management are used independent of the skill of the rescuer, and have become ubiquitous in both pediatric and adult, and basic to advanced life support training. (**Ref. 12,** p. 112)

24. **(C)** Airway control in the traumatized patient is performed to protect or provide a patent airway. Airway patency may be lost when brain injury or intoxication result in loss of protective reflexes such as gag, when the airway has been traumatized, or when foreign material is present in the oropharynx and the patient cannot clear it. This patient's head injury has resulted in altered mental status which may impede his ability to protect his own airway and is an indication for tracheal intubation. Similarly, blood, tooth fragments, vomit, or swelling may obstruct the patient's airway. Upper airway noise relieved with jaw thrust suggests that protective reflexes may already be lost. Lack of breath sounds on auscultation without other evidence of respiratory compromise is not an indication for intubation. (**Ref. 12,** p. 277)

25. **(B)** By definition, a pneumothorax is entrance of air into the pleural space during inspiration. In simple pneumothorax, there is entrance of air through the parenchymal pleura with no associated mediastinal shift or elevated intrapleural pressure. Communicating pneumothorax has free communication of air through the chest wall. In both simple and communicating pneumothorax, there is equalization of pleural and atmospheric pressure. Tension pneumothorax is due to the inability to equalize pressures between the pleural space and the atmosphere when a defect in the pleura allows air entrance to the pleural space on inspiration, but not exit on expiration. Tension pneumothorax causes a breath by breath

hyperexpansion of the pleural space on the affected side. The resultant mediastinal shift and elevated intrathoracic pressure causes decreased venous return and hypotension. A hemodynamically significant tension pneumothorax requires immediate needle or tube thoracostomy to decompress the chest to allow for equalization of atmospheric and pleural pressures. (**Ref. 12,** pp. 433–436)

26. **(D)**   The single most common cause of hypotension in the traumatized patient is hypovolemia due to hemorrhage. However, hypotension is not the only manifestation of shock. Tachycardia, altered mental status ranging from anxiety to coma, slowed capillary refill, and pallor and diaphoresis occur according to the degree of shock. Hypotension due to intracranial injury, spinal shock, intoxication, or cardiac contusion may occur in the traumatized patient. However, hypovolemia must be excluded as the primary cause before these diagnoses are considered solely. (**Ref. 12,** pp. 268–269)

27. **(A)**   The fluid resuscitation of the patient with hypovolemic shock due to hemorrhage represents an ongoing controversy. However, the most well accepted management strategy consists of infusion of isosmotic crystalloid rapidly and continuous reassessment of response. If the desired hemodynamic response does not occur, then O negative or cross-matched blood is given. Withholding fluid replacement and using vasopressor agents in the management of hemorrhagic shock is not acceptable management. Hypertonic crystalloid with dextran is under trial, and has shown benefit over isosmotic crystalloid in improving blood pressure in the hypovolemic patient. Finally, colloid infusion is more expensive than crystalloid, and has never been shown to be of benefit in resuscitation. (**Ref. 12,** p. 168)

28. **(A)**   The presentation of a new diabetic with ketoacidosis is most consistent with Type I diabetes mellitus. These patients have insulin lack which is characterized by near absence or total absence of the C-peptide fraction of the insulin molecule. The ketones in the urine are those with carboxyl or ketone groups attached, acetoacetate, and acetone. Beta hydroxybutyrate does not show up on a typical urine dip stick. Insulin resistance is more a component of

Type II diabetes mellitus and is unlikely to play a role in this case. A family history of Type I diabetes mellitus is unusual as the occurrence of diabetes in these patients tends to be more sporadic than familial. (**Ref. 1,** pp. 190–193)

29. **(B)** The mainstay of treating diabetic acidosis is infusion of isotonic fluid, typically saline, plus the administration of insulin. In this patient, who is mildly hypokalemic, it is reasonable to give potassium early in the management. Aggressive replacement of sodium bicarbonate may cause the patient to become rapidly alkalotic, which may have a detrimental effect on the oxygen delivery to tissues. (**Ref. 1,** p. 1992)

30. **(C)** The hallmark of cardiac tamponade is the paradoxical pulse which is also seen in constrictive pericarditis, hypovolemic shock, severe asthma, or COPD. Critical aortic stenosis is associated with a narrowed pulse pressure. Acute myocardial infarction may lead to a thready pulse, but is not associated with a paradoxic pulse. Pulmonary embolism can lead to a marked sensation of dyspnea and may be associated with enhanced right-sided heart sounds, but is not typically associated with paradox pulse. (**Ref. 1,** p. 1097)

31. **(B)** A careful history and physical examination are clearly the most useful diagnostic tests to evaluate patients with syncope; the yield of other tests is much lower. Twenty-four-hour ambulatory ECG monitoring and intracardiac electrophysiologic evaluation with programmed atrial ventricular stimulation may detect cardiac arrhythmias as the cause of otherwise unexplained syncope, especially if the syncope is recurrent, or the patient has structural heart disease. In patients with recurrent syncope of unknown cause, the long-term prognosis is excellent. In patients with a documented cardiac cause of syncope, the incidence of sudden death after one year is approximately 25%. Despite extensive evaluation, no diagnosis is made in more than 50% of patients with syncope. (**Ref. 22,** pp. 879–885)

32. **(A)** Of the valve lesions listed, only hypertrophic obstructive cardiomyopathy, also known as subaortic stenosis, is associated with a murmur that increases in intensity upon standing up. Presumably, the decrease in filling pressure of the left ventricle narrows the aortic outflow track and leads to an enhancement and prolongation of the murmur. Diminished flow rates through the aortic and mitral valve lead to a decrease in the murmurs associated with aortic stenosis, mitro regurgitation, and atrial septal defect. Aortic regurgitation is a diastolic murmur. (**Ref. 1**, p. 1092)

33. **(B)** New onset of generalized or localized seizures in persons who are over 50 years of age most commonly results from cerebral vascular disease, especially as a late sequel to cerebral thrombosis, embolus, or hemorrhage. Less frequently, these disorders may present acutely with a seizure. Brain tumors are the second most common cause of seizures in this age group. In young adults aged 18 to 35, prior head trauma, alcoholism, and brain tumors are the most common causes of seizures. (**Ref. 1**, pp. 22–27)

34. **(D)** The pH shows that the primary process is an acidosis. The PCO2 shows that there is hyperventilation to compensate. The anion gap is calculated to be 20; therefore, this is an increased anion gap acidosis with respiratory compensation suggesting this is primarily a metabolic acidosis. (**Ref. 1**, p. 255)

35. **(D)** The anion gap acidoses include diabetic ketoacidosis, alcoholic ketoacidosis, ingestion, renal failure, and sepsis. Diarrhea, renal tubular acidosis, etc. lead to a non-anion gap acidosis. Anxiety, mechanical ventilation, etc. lead to primary respiratory alkalosis. Hepatic cirrhosis, pregnancy, and cerebral disease all can lead to chronic respiratory alkalosis with metabolic compensation. (**Ref. 1**, pp. 256–257)

36. **(B)** In keeping with the differential diagnosis outlined in the previous question, the diagnostic tests of choice would look at the presence of diabetes, the presence of renal insufficiency, and the presence of unmeasured anions. The urine pH, stool electrolytes, and calcium would be measures of things that could lead to a non-

anion gap acidosis. Serum ammonias and CAT scan of the head would address the issue of primary chronic respiratory alkalosis. (**Ref. 1**, pp. 256–257)

37. (**A**) Pupillary dilation, not constriction, is usually seen during or shortly after use. In addition to the symptoms listed, elevated or lowered blood pressure, evidence of weight loss, perspiration or chills, muscular weakness, respiratory depression, chest pains, cardiac arrthythmias, confusion, seizures, dyskinesias, dystonias, or coma may accompany amphetamine use. (**Ref. 10**, pp. 411–416)

38. (**E**) Upper airway obstruction, caused by inflammatory processes, results in more symptomatology in children than in adults due to the smaller pediatric airway. While the majority of inflammatory processes causing upper airway obstruction are viral in origin, differentiating between the viral disease, laryngotracheobronchitis (croup), and bacterial processes is made more important by the increased risk of complete obstruction seen in bacterial epiglottitis and/or tracheitis. Historical information can often assist in the differentiation of bacterial vs. viral etiologies. Croup is usually preceded by an upper respiratory tract infection followed by the onset of a barky cough. Fever may be low-grade or can achieve levels of 40°C. When calm, most children with croup appear relatively well with minimal distress. In the presence of upper airway obstruction of any cause, agitation and crying may increase stridor due to increased air flow past the obstruction. (**Ref. 5**, pp. 1201–1208)

39. (**B**) Children with bacterial etiologies often have a more abrupt onset, higher fevers, appear toxic, and may drool or develop aphonia. The progression of this disease is often rapid and can result in complete obstruction and death if treatment is not initiated. Fixed obstruction due to subglottic stenosis may also result in stridor. The most common cause of chronic subglottic stenosis is neonatal intubation. (**Ref. 5**, pp. 1201–1208)

40. (**D**) Evaluation of any patient with evidence of upper airway obstruction includes assessment of air entry (breath sounds), evaluation of the work of breathing (respiratory rate and the presence or absence of retractions), and observation of adequacy of oxygenation (cyanosis and oxygen saturation). In the presence of significant stridor, invasive procedures such as blood gases and use of a tongue depressor should be deferred until the airway has improved. The lateral neck radiograph is often normal in croup, but identifies edema of the epiglottis in children with epiglottitis and may demonstrate strandy membranes in children with bacterial tracheitis. Inspiratory and expiratory chest films are useful when evaluating for a foreign body but will most likely not assist in the diagnosis of croup or epiglottitis. (**Ref. 5,** pp. 1201–1208)

41. (**C**) Laryngotracheobronchitis (croup) is the most common etiology resulting in upper airway obstruction. Seventy-five percent of cases are the result of infection with the parainfluenza viruses although adenovirus and influenza virus have been known to cause croup. Prior to the Hib vaccine, hemophilus influenzae, type B, was the most frequent etiology in patients with epiglottitis. Epiglottitis has also been associated with *Streptococcus pneumoniae*. Bacterial tracheitis is often a secondary infection and is frequently caused by *Staphylococcus aureus*. (**Ref. 5,** pp. 1201–1208)

42. (**E**) The treatment of croup depends on the symptoms of the patients. Many patients with mild symptoms (cough and low grade fever) can be cared for at home. Evidence of increased airway obstruction often results in hospital admission. Humidified air will often decrease respiratory distress and laryngospasm within minutes of use. This may be due to the cooling effect which results in decreases in edema. Antipyretics will decrease fever when present, decreasing metabolic rate and, potentially, the respiratory rate. Careful observation of the degree of airway obstruction is necessary. The use of steroids is controversial with some literature supporting their use while other studies demonstrate no advantage. The use of antibiotics in patients with viral disease is not indicated. Racemic epinephrine is useful in transiently improving airway obstruction, but close observation and, potentially, repeated administration may be necessary. (**Ref. 5,** pp. 1201–1208)

43. (D); 44. (D); 45. (B); 46. (E); 47. (B)   Asthma is the most common chronic illness of childhood and is responsible for more unplanned pediatric hospital admissions than any other disease. The majority of children (80% to 90%) are symptomatic by age 4 to 5 years. However, the progression of disease varies tremendously with some children having minimal symptoms and impact, to others with severe disease associated with lost school days, increased use of medical resources and, occasionally, mortality. The symptoms of asthma are the result of inflammation of the airways compounded by bronchoconstriction. Triggers may include exposure to inhaled allergens (pollens, dust mites, pet dander), environmental pollutants (smoke, air pollutants), cold air, excercise, or emotional events. The usual treatment includes avoidance of triggers, beta adrenergic agents, and chromolyn sodium. Acute exacerbations require increased frequency of treatment and, often, oxygen supplementation and steroids.

The goal of long-term management is to provide appropriate treatment based on frequent assessment of pulmonary function. The use of peak flow meters and individualized crisis management allow the child and family to intervene early, often preventing progression of the disease and the need for additional evaluation. This will also allow maintenance of functional behavior. Asthma is the cause of significant loss of school days and the loss of work days for caretakers. While changes in the home and social environment may alter compliance and result in (transient) changes in disease severity, the functional impact can best be assessed by school absences and performance.

When home management fails, children often require treatment in an acute care setting such as the ED. The severity of disease can be estimated using objective criteria such as expiratory peak flow, heart rate, respiratory rate, and oxygen saturation as well as findings from the clinical exam which identify increased work of breathing or dyspnea. Peak expiratory flow rates of > 70% predicted are evidence of a mild exacerbation, while levels < 50% predicted indicate a severe exacerbation. The mild hyperventilation often seen in a mild, acute exacerbation results in hypocapnia. Normal or elevated CO_2 levels are indicative of moderate and severe exacerbations respectively. Markedly increased respiratory rates also occur with severe exacerbations although mild elevations may be seen even in mild disease. Wheezing is present even in mild exacerbations while inaudible breath sounds suggest a severe exacerbation. Dyspnea can also be used to assess severity, while breathlessness and inability to speak in full sentences indicates high severity.

Inpatient management of asthma includes beta adrenergic therapy, either by inhalation or IV administration. Directed at the relief of bronchospasm, these agents also result in pulmonary vasodilation. In the normal pulmonary vascular bed, local hypoxia, such as that which occurs in atelectasis, results in pulmonary vasoconstriction in an effort to preserve ventilation-perfusion matching. The beta agonists blunt the normal vasoconstriction and may result in worsening of V/Q matching leading to hypoxemia during administration of these agents. (**Ref. 5,** pp. 628–640)

4

Satellite Health Center

DIRECTIONS (Questions 1–38): Each of the numbered items or incomplete statements in this chapter is followed by answers or completions of the statement. Select the **ONE** lettered answer or completion that is **BEST** in each case.

1. During a routine visit to the clinic, Sara's mother raises the question of screening for lead poisoning. Sara is a healthy 5-year-old with a normal physical exam. She attends a local kindergarten. The historical information which would put Sara at low risk for lead poisoning is

    A. the family lives near Sara's father place of employment, a foundry which recycles batteries

    B. the family's home was built in 1980 and they recently began renovating the kitchen

    C. several of Sara's classmates have recently been treated for elevated lead levels

    D. Sara's lead level when she was 36 months was 15 micrograms/deciliter

    E. Sara's mother enjoys making pottery and uses a variety of foreign glazes

2. A 10-month-old black male is brought to the clinic with rhinorrhea, congestion, and fever. On physical examination the child has nasal congestion and an erythematous right typmanic membrane. The appropriate next diagnostic study is

   A. pneumatic otoscopy

   B. tympanocentesis

   C. nasopharyngeal culture

   D. tympanometry

   E. no further studies are required

3. A 3-year-old with a 1 cm honey-colored crusted lesion on the right knee has been brought to the office. You diagnose impetigo and begin appropriate antibiotic therapy. You provide appropriate discharge instructions directed at possible complications. The most likely complication from impetigo is

   A. acute glomerulonephritis

   B. septicemia

   C. osteomyelitis

   D. cellulitis

   E. suppurative lymphadenitis

4. A 16-year-old with dysuria arrives at the clinic with her mother. While her mother is out of the room, she confides that she may have "gotten something" from her boyfriend. She admits that she has been sexually active for the last year. She believes her mother is unaware of this and asks you not to say anything since if her mother knew "she would kill me." You perform the appropriate diagnostic tests. The appropriate next step is to

   A. ask the mother to return to the room and discuss the patient's sexual activity and need for contraception with both present

   B. inform the girl that, since she is a minor, you will disclose her sexual activity to her mother once she is asked back into the room

C. ask the mother to return to the room but say nothing about the discussion the 16-year-old had with you in private

D. encourage your patient to reveal her activities to her mother, then ask the mother to return to the room to discuss the treatment plan, revealing nothing of your discussion with the 16-year-old

E. call Child Protection Services to report the statutory rape of this minor

5. During a sports physical examination for a basketball camp, a 15-year-old asks you about the growth shots he has heard about. His dream is to be a professional basketball player. He is at the 65th percentile for height and has been growing normally. His father is 5'10" and his mother is 5'6". His sexual maturation rating is Tanner stage 4. The appropriate next step is

A. obtain blood levels of growth hormone to determine whether he is deficient

B. assure him that he will achieve sufficient height to play professional basketball

C. explain that exogenous growth hormone is ineffective in achieving additional growth in people with normal growth hormone levels

D. assure him that he has constitutional growth delay and will experience "catch-up" growth soon

E. explain that growth hormone would be unlikely to produce added height in him, but that he will continue to grow over the next several years

6. A 5-year-old is brought to the clinic for evaluation of puffiness around the eyes. He was well until two weeks ago, when he had a mild cold. His cold symptoms improved but now he has swelling around the eyes, especially in the morning. He has had no fever, no significant change in urinary or bowel habits, and no change in the color of his urine. His appetite is somewhat decreased. His laboratory results reveal the following:

Urinalysis: specific gravity: 1.025 protein: 4+ 0-3 WBC/HPF
            blood: negative   2-5 RBC/HPF
            glucose: negative

Chemistries: glucose: 90mg/dL   albumin: 2.4mg/dL
            cholesterol: 405 mM/L triglycerides: 185 mg/dL

The most likely etiology for this disease is

A. focal glomerulosclerosis

B. membranoproliferative disease

C. minimal change disease

D. mesangial proliferative disease

E. post-streptococcal glomerulonephritis

Case Cluster (Questions 7–9):

7. A 21-year-old female college student comes into the student health service where you work part-time requesting evaluation of pharyngitis. History of present illness is remarkable for two-day history of fatigue, fever to 101, anorexia, and severe throat pain. Her physical exam reveals a temperature of 100.1, tender enlarged anterior cervical nodes, and large red tonsils with exudate. "Rapid strep" is positive for strep. The preferred therapy for strep pharyngitis is

A. pen VK 250 mg tid × 10 days

B. benzathine penicillin 1.2 million units IM given once

C. pen VK 500 mg qid 1 week

D. erythromycin 250 mg qid × 10 days

E. pen VK 500 mg bid × 10d

8. Because you realize that college students don't usually come in for regular health maintenance visits, you decide to offer some prevention at this "acute care" visit. The important clinical prevention strategies in her age group would include all of the following **EXCEPT**

   A. education and counseling regarding alcohol, tobacco, and other drug abuse and use

   B. cholesterol check

   C. breast cancer screening

   D. immunization for hepatitis

   E. immunization for measles

9. She tells you she has never been sexually active and has no plans to become sexually active in the near future, therefore, does not want a Pap smear and pelvic exam. You tell her

   A. she does not need a Pap smear until she becomes sexually active as long as she has no gynecological problems or abnormalities

   B. all women over 18 years of age should get a yearly Pap smear and pelvic examination

   C. she needs a pelvic examination but does not need a Pap smear or vaginal cultures

   D. all women of reproductive age need gynecological examination once a year

   E. all women from the onset of menses until 65 to 70 years of age need a yearly pelvic examination

Case Cluster (Questions 10–13):

10. A young female college student asks your opinion regarding oral contraceptive pills, which she is considering starting. You explain that contraindication to oral contraceptive pills include all the following **EXCEPT**

    A. impaired liver function

    B. smoker and aged over 35 years

    C. thromboembolic disease

    D. diabetes

    E. systemic lupus erythematosis

11. You explain to her that relative contraindications to using oral contraceptives include all of the following **EXCEPT**

    A. history of migraines

    B. hypertension

    C. diabetes

    D. sickle cell anemia

    E. iron deficiency anemia

12. You also tell her that it is important to consider the many benefits of oral contraceptive pills. Oral contraceptives have been shown to decrease hospitalizations for all of the following conditions **EXCEPT**

    A. ectopic pregnancy

    B. ovarian cysts

    C. endometrial cancer

D. pelvic inflammatory disease

E. breast cancer

13. Other benefits to consider include all of the following **EXCEPT**

    A. less vaso-occlusive pain crises from sickle cell disease

    B. lighter and less painful menses

    C. improvement in iron deficiency anemia

    D. decreased incidence of pelvic inflammatory disease

    E. an improvement in hirsutism

Case Cluster (Questions 14–15):

14. You are counseling a young woman with a recently diagnosed breast mass and needle biopsy proven cancer. Regarding her potential survival based on mastectomy findings, the most true statement is

    A. survival is inversely proportional to the number of affected regional lymph nodes

    B. tumor size does not correlate with the expected number of positive nodes

    C. node negative and node positive patients have an equal likelihood of distant metastasis

    D. node negative and node positive patients have an equal likelihood of disease relapse

    E. distant metastasis does not correlate with survival

15. Which of the following is **NOT** a risk factor for the development of breast cancer?

A. High fat diet

B. Obesity

C. Infertility or nulliparity

D. Combined oral contraceptives

E. Family history of breast cancer in first degree relatives

16. A 42-year-old man presents to the clinic with the complaint of "tongue swelling and difficulty swallowing." A friend accompanies the patient and tells you that these symptoms began the prior evening after a one-week history of toothache. Examination reveals the patient to be febrile, with tense swelling in the submandibular area pushing the tongue posterior and cephalad. He is drooling, dysphonic, and has trismus which limits your posterior pharynx examination. The most likely diagnosis in this patient is

A. angioedema

B. buccal cellulitis

C. periapical abscess

D. Ludwig's angina

E. peritonsillar abscess

17. A patient presents to the clinic with the complaint of a persistent nosebleed for two hours. Which of the following statements about epistaxis is **INCORRECT**?

  A. Posterior epistaxis is more common in the elderly, and in patients with uncontrolled hypertension

  B. Posterior nasal packing, while uncomfortable, is a relatively benign procedure with little comorbidity

  C. Patients with nasal packing in place should be given prophylactic antibiotics

  D. Bleeding from Kisselbach's plexus in an uncomplicated patient may be controlled with direct pressure to the nasal septum for 10 minutes

  E. Anterior bleeding which is recurrent or uncontrolled requires an anterior nasal pack

18. A patient presents to your office with the complaint of rectal pain. The **INCORRECT** statement regarding anorectal complaints is

  A. internal hemorrhoids frequently cause rectal bleeding without pain

  B. external hemorrhoids frequently cause rectal pain without bleeding

  C. anal fissures frequently cause rectal bleeding without pain

  D. anorectal abscesses frequently cause rectal pain without bleeding

  E. diverticulosis frequently causes rectal bleeding without pain

19. A 30-year-old white male presents to an urgent care clinic with a severe, penetrating pain behind the right eye associated with tearing and nasal stuffiness. This intense headache has occurred each of the last three nights, waking him at approximately 1 a.m. and lasting two to three hours. This is most likely

   A. migraine headache

   B. tension headache

   C. increased intracranial pressure

   D. cluster headache

   E. sinus headache

20. A 20-year-old black male presents to the student health service with severe tenosynovitis at the wrist and ankles. Physical examination reveals oral ulcerations, balanitis, and a thick scaly rash on the palms and soles. This is most likely associated with

   A. gonococcemia

   B. *Chlamydia trachomatis*

   C. psoriasis

   D. beta-hemolytic streptococcus

   E. syphilis

21. A 45-year-old Hispanic man, treated for deep venous thrombosis, presents to an urgent care center with a severe nosebleed. The prothrombin time is markedly elevated at 45 seconds (INR = 8.5). Which of these components of the history might explain the problem?

   A. Recent increase in smoking from one to two packs per day

   B. Recent diagnosis of increased cholesterol with initiation of cholestyramine therapy

   C. Recent bronchitis treated with trimethoprim/sulfamethoxazole

   D. A recent change in diet emphasizing green vegetables

   E. Non-compliance with his medication, frequently skipping doses

22. A line worker in an auto factory presents to the company doctor with acute back pain after trying to prevent an engine block from slipping off a hoist. Examination reveals marked paraspinous muscle spasm, a positive straight leg raising test, and an absent ankle jerk. The most likely diagnosis is

   A. acute muscle strain

   B. L-4 nerve root irritation

   C. S-1 herniated disc with nerve root compression

   D. L-3 herniated disc with nerve root compression

   E. compression fracture of L-5

Case Cluster (Questions 23–28):

23. A 26-year-old married Catholic female graduate student presents to the student health service complaining of problems sleeping. Upon further questioning you elicit a history of early morning awakening, seven pound weight loss, decreased sexual drive, and difficulty concentrating. You consider asking about suicidal thoughts. Which of the following statements is true about suicidal ideation?

    A. Broaching the question plants the seed

    B. Her religion will prevent her from taking any action

    C. People who talk about it, won't do it

    D. She may be relieved to be able to discuss these feelings

    E. Marriage protects

24. Which of the following is the most likely diagnosis?

    A. Major depressive disorder

    B. Major depressive disorder with melancholic features

    C. Dysthymic disorder

    D. Bipolar disorder, most recent episode depressed

    E. Cyclothymic cisorder

25. The **LEAST** important factor that may influence your choice of antidepressant therapy is

    A. other concurrent medications

    B. efficacy

C. side effects

D. half-life

E. cost

26. You decide to choose a selective serotonin reuptake inhibitor (SSRI). The following SSRI dosage ranges are correct **EXCEPT**

A. Sertraline (Zoloft) 50 to 200 mg/day

B. Paroxetine (Paxil) 10 to 50 mg/day

C. Fluoxetine (Prozac) 20 to 80 mg/day

D. Fluvoxamine (Luvox) 150 to 300 mg/day

E. Clomipramine (Anafranil) 10 to 50 mg/day

27. The woman returns to your office reporting considerable improvement of her depressive symptoms over the past month after taking the medication you prescribed. The one symptom that has not improved is her sexual drive. She continues to have no interest in sex. Prior to her depressive episode, she and her husband had sexual intercourse two or three time a week. The most likely cause of her sexual difficulties is

A. her depressive symptoms have not completely resolved yet

B. she has marital difficulties of which she has not informed you

C. her antidepressant medication may be the cause

D. she may be entering her monthly menstrual cycle

E. she may be starting menopause

28. Selective serotonin reuptake inhibitors (SSRI's) have been increasingly used because of all of the following reasons **EXCEPT**

    A. less expensive

    B. less anticholinergic

    C. less cardiotoxic

    D. less sedation

    E. equally effective

29. A 27-year-old businessman presents to your downtown clinic complaining of nasal congestion and nose bleeds. Physical examination reveals inflammation and ulceration of the nasal mucosa as well as perforation of the nasal septa. Associated conditions may include all of the following **EXCEPT**

    A. nonhemorrhagic cerebral infarctions

    B. seizures

    C. arrhythmias

    D. death

    E. liver disease

30. One January day, a pharmaceutical representative drops by your satellite clinic in northern Wisconsin to inform you of a medical conference in San Diego, California in three weeks that would update you on an important new product. If you can take the time off, his company will fly you and your spouse to the meeting, provide three nights lodging, and cover your meals for the trip. Your best option is

    A. go home and discuss the offer with your spouse

    B. politely refuse the invitation

    C. check your schedule and check departure times

D. accept the invitation

E. consult with your clinic's legal counsel

Case Cluster (Questions 31–33):

31. During a preemployment physical examination, a 29-year-old single black male reveals to you that he has experienced bouts of depression in each of the last three winters. Symptoms include difficulty concentrating, early morning awakening, and loss of appetite. He has had some thoughts during these periods that he would be better off dead, but he has never done anything about them. Between these episodes he has been doing well and reports no problems. He has never seen a psychiatrist. He had no positive findings on physical exam and denies any medication use, prescribed or otherwise. Your most likely diagnosis should be

   A. bipolar I disorder

   B. schizoaffective disorder

   C. major depressive disorder with seasonal pattern

   D. cyclothymic disorder

   E. substance-induced mood disorder

32. Treatment for this condition could include all of the following **EXCEPT**

   A. tricyclic antidepressants

   B. phototherapy

   C. selective serotonin reuptake inhibitors

   D. electroconvulsive therapy

   E. anticonvulsant therapy

33. Factors associated with efficacy of phototherapy include all of the following **EXCEPT**

    A. high intensity light is better than dim light

    B. shorter duration appears more effective

    C. timing of treatments is important

    D. eye exposure is more effective than skin exposure

    E. spectral quality may be a factor

Case Cluster (Questions 34–38):

34. Recently a new family with three children entered your practice. The oldest child is a 7-year-old boy who has been healthy except for frequent ear infections in the first year of life. The second child is 4 years old and has trisomy 21. She has been hospitalized several times, first for congestive heart failure due to an endocardial cushion defect (with an abnormal valve) and subsequently for RSV bronchiolitis and frequent respiratory infections. The youngest child is 10 months old and has been healthy. The family's fourth child is due in a week or so. The mother brings the 7-year-old boy to the office for evaluation of bedwetting. He had not wet the bed since he was four or so, but has recently begun having "accidents" several times each week. Mom has tried punishing him for these events but it has not helped. Physical examination and evaluation reveal a healthy 7-year-old. The appropriate advice to provide is

    A. tell the child that he should not be wetting the bed and should drink less prior to bedtime

    B. reassure the mother that many 7-year-old boys still have enuresis and that it will go away with time

    C. prescribe a short period of DDAVP to break the cycle of enuresis

D. explain that her son has secondary enuresis, possibly due to the stress of the new baby, and it should be transient

E. encourage negative reinforcement for each episode to decrease the incidence of enuresis

35. The mother begins to discuss the care of the 4-year-old. Up to this point the child has received no immunizations since she was "sick all the time." The child has been well for the last year or so and Mom wants to begin immunizations today. In addition to polio vaccination, the appropriate set of immunizations to order is

A. DTP, Hib, MMR

B. DTP, Hepatovax, MMR

C. DT, Hib, Hepatovax, MMR

D. Td, Hib, Hepatovax, MMR

E. DTP, Hib, Hepatovax, MMR

36. After the discussion about vaccinations, Mom asks you about the growth pattern of her 4-year-old child. She is quite a bit shorter than her brother was at the same age and seems to grow somewhat slower as well. On plotting the child's height and weight she is just below the fifth percentile for weight but considerably below the fifth percentile for height. The next appropriate step is

A. obtain a bone age to determine whether there is delay in bone maturation

B. replot the measurements using a chart designed for children with trisomy 21

C. obtain growth hormone levels to evaluate for possible deficiency

D. measure thyroid hormone levels for possible hyperthyroidism

E. suggest that Mom obtain previous growth records and begin a calorie count at home

37. The family is also concerned about the long-term problems their child with trisomy 21 may experience. You explain that patients with trisomy 21 are at increased risk for all of the following **EXCEPT**

    A. accelerated atherosclerotic heart disease

    B. leukemia

    C. diabetes

    D. cataract

    E. Alzheimer's disease

38. During the exam of the 4-year-old, you notice poor dentition. Your refer the child for further evaluation by a pediatric dentist. The next appropriate step is

    A. arrange for an exam under anesthesia as the child is not likely to hold still

    B. discuss the need for probable orthodontic surgery as children with trisomy 21 have an increased risk of caries

    C. describe the expected procedures to the child to prepare her for the visit in three weeks

    D. discuss the importance of not using a bottle at night to avoid further problems with "baby bottle tooth decay"

    E. prescribe prophylactic antibiotics for use prior to and after the dental exam

Satellite Health Center

Answers and Discussion

1. **(B)** Lead poisoning is defined as having a lead level of 10 micrograms/dL or more. Risk factors for children 6 months to 6 years of age include: living in a home built before 1960 that is in poor condition or undergoing renovation, having siblings or playmates with known lead poisoning, having a family member who participates in a lead-related hobby or job, or living near industries which release atmospheric lead, including battery recycling plants. (**Ref. 6**, pp. 16–17)

2. **(A)** The diagnosis of otitis media can be made by visualization of an erythematous tympanic membrane. However, since crying may result in hyperemia of the TM, pneumatic otoscopy should reveal a nonmobile tympanic membrane before the diagnosis is made. Tympanocentesis will provide a specimen for identification of a causal agent when the diagnosis is doubtful or when the patient is seriously ill, is failing to respond to treatment, or is receiving antibiotics when they develop the otitis. (**Ref. 5**, pp. 1814–1817)

3. **(D)** The predominant organism causing impetigo is *Staphylococcus aureus* with group A β hemolytic streptococci being responsible for some lesions. Septicemia, osteomyelitis, and suppurative lymphadenitis are potential complications from lesions caused by either organism while acute glomerulonephritis occurs

151

after infection with group A β hemolytic streptococci. However, cellulitis is the most frequent complication, occurring in 10% of patients with nonbullous impetigo (the type described here). (**Ref. 5,** p. 1890)

4. **(D)** The patient-physician interaction is delicate at any time, but at no time is it more difficult that with a teen who could be considered emancipated. Discussing the child's sexual activity after her explicit request not to is a breach of confidentiality. (**Ref. 6,** pp. 80–81)

5. **(E)** For the otherwise healthy individual, determination of final adult height is a combination of genetics and nutrition. A young man at the 65th percentile does not meet criteria for growth failure unless prior growth was at a substantially higher percentile. Therefore, measurement of growth hormone levels would be unnecessary (and expensive). Given the height of his parents, it does not appear that he is experiencing constitutional growth delay either. This patient will benefit from an explanation of his expected growth over the next several years as well as a discussion about the inability to increase his final adult height by administering exogenous growth hormone. (**Ref. 6,** pp. 1687–1693)

6. **(C)** Nephrotic syndrome is produced by massive loss of protein in the urine. The loss of predominantly albumin leads to a decrease in oncotic pressure and development of edema. In addition, elevation of serum cholesterol and triglycerides are seen. The most frequent etiology for nephrotic syndrome in children is minimal change disease. The morphology of the glomeruli appears normal on light microscopy. However, electron microscopy reveals fusion of the epithelial cell podocytes. Membranoproliferative disease, focal glomerulosclerosis, and mesangial proliferative disease all can result in nephrotic syndrome but are far less common as the etiology. Post streptococcal glomerulonephritis, an immunologically mediated disease, presents with edema, hematuria and, in some patients, hypertension. Although hypoproteinemia and elevated serum lipids can occur, these are unusual in PSGN. (**Ref. 6,** pp. 1366–1367, 1352–1353)

7. **(B)** Strep pharyngitis can often resolve spontaneously on its own. Treatment of strep pharyngitis is aimed at reducing symptoms more quickly. In addition, treatment with antibiotics also decreases the incidence of complications such as peritonsillar abscess and rheumatic heart fever. Parental therapy with 1.2 million units of benzathine penicillin is the preferred method of treatment because of compliance issues. Only a ten-day course of oral antibiotic has been shown to affect the incidence of rheumatic heart disease. However, penicillin and erythromycin can be dosed in any of the ways listed as long as the total course is at least ten days. IM benzathine penicillin is also effective. (**Ref. 20,** p. 334)

8. **(C)** In the periodic health examination or urgent care visits, clinical prevention strategies should target common, age-specific, and preventable conditions. In adolescents and young adults, immunization for hepatitis and measles is a cost-effective method for reducing the incidence of these conditions. Detecting and then reducing elevated cholesterol by diet, exercise, or medication can effectively decrease heart disease in later years. Substance abuse and smoking often begin in adolescence or early adulthood. Education and counseling can help prevent the initiation of these habits or get people to stop before they suffer the consequences. Breast cancer is extremely rare in young adulthood and detection with mammography or self breast exam does not lead to improved long-term outcomes. (**Ref. 20,** p. 20)

9. **(B)** Pelvic examination is aimed at detecting cervical cancer, sexually transmitted diseases, or other gynecological problems as well as pregnancy. If a patient has not been sexually active, she is not at risk for sexually transmitted diseases. Although cervical cancer has been linked to human papilloma virus infection which is also sexually transmitted, Pap smears can detect other cervical dysplasias. Good scientific evidence exists to support recommending yearly pelvic exams with Pap smears to women beginning at age 18 or at onset of sexual activity. Gynecological tumors, ovarian and endometrial cancers can occur in older women. Because the incidence in women over age 65 greatly diminishes, pelvic exams after age 65 become less important as a prevention strategy. (**Ref. 20,** p. 20)

10. (D) Women who have diabetes can use oral contraceptives although some may require an adjustment of their insulin dose. Absolute contraindications to contraceptives include impaired liver function (until LFTs return to normal), gall bladder disease, thromboembolic disease including cerebrovascular events, as well as hyperlipidemia, myocardial infarction, pregnancy, or smokers who are over 35 years of age. (**Ref. 9**, p. 745)

11. (E) In menstruating females, iron deficiency anemia is usually caused by a combination of poor diet and heavy menstrual bleeding. Since oral contraceptives usually lighten menstrual flow, they usually improve anemia when menstruation is part of its cause. All of the other conditions listed have been impacted unfavorably by oral contraceptives. (**Ref. 9**, p. 746)

12. (E) Because the link between breast cancer and oral contraceptives is still controversial, it is advisable not to prescribe them in cases of known or suspected breast cancer. However, oral contraceptives have been shown to decrease hospitalizations due to ectopic pregnancy, ovarian cancer, endometrial cancer, and pelvic inflammatory disease. (**Ref. 9**, p. 745)

13. (A) Oral contraceptives can theoretically cause vaso-occlusive crises in sickle cell anemia. However, it is often worth a trial of their use because many patients with sickle cell can use them as effective contraception without increased pain crises. (**Ref. 9**, p. 744)

14. (A) The likelihood of survival in breast cancer is inversely proportional to the number of positive lymph nodes. Larger tumor size correlates with the likelihood of positive nodes. Node positive patients have a higher likelihood of both distant metastasis and relapse. Finally, more than 95% of patients who die of breast cancer have distant metastasis. (**Ref. 14**, p. 556)

15. (D) High fat diet, obesity, infertility, and nulliparity increase the risk of breast cancer. Early age of first pregnancy is relatively protective. Breast feeding and combined oral contraceptives appear to have no net positive or negative effect on the risk of developing breast cancer. (**Ref. 14,** p. 553)

16. **(D)** Ludwig's angina is defined as bilateral submandibular cellulitis. It usually originates from an odontogenic infection, and results in the physical findings described. This patient should be admitted to an intensive care unit for close observation, as laryngospasm is a frequent complication of Ludwig's angina. Approximately one-third of patients require intubation or tracheostomy. Angioedema, buccal abscess, periapical abscess, and peritonsillar abscess are unlikely to cause isolated swelling of the submandibular region. Angioedema and peritonsillar abscess are unlikely to present in association with an odontogenic infection. However, peritonsillar abscess may cause trismus, dysphonia, and drooling. (**Ref. 15,** pp. 1077–1080)

17. **(B)** Epistaxis is divided by origin into anterior and posterior. Anterior bleeding generally occurs from Kisselbach's plexus on the anterior, inferior septum, and may usually be controlled by direct pressure. Recurrent or uncontrolled anterior bleeding, and all posterior bleeding will require nasal packing. Anterior packing is relatively benign, but does place the patient at risk for sinusitis and toxic shock syndrome. Thus patients with nasal packs should be treated with prophylactic antibiotics. Patients with posterior nasal packs are at risk for hypoventilation and hypercarbia, and accidental dislodgement of the pack into the posterior pharynx. All patients with posterior packing, especially those who have chronic obstructive pulmonary disease, should be considered candidates for hospital admission and observation. (**Ref. 15,** pp. 1082–1087)

18. **(C)** Internal hemorrhoids and diverticulosis usually cause rectal bleeding without pain. External hemorrhoids usually cause rectal pain without bleeding. Anal fissures, however, cause both pain and bleeding, and are usually caused by sharp or large stools. The fissure most often develops at the posterior midline of the anus. Chronic fissures have an internal hypertrophied papilla, a shallow

ulcer just inside the anal verge, and a tag of hypertrophied skin externally referred to as a sentinel pile. Stool softeners, Sitz baths, and topical anesthetics are used for control of symptoms, with most fissures healing spontaneously. (**Ref. 12,** pp. 1661–1663)

19. **(D)** Headaches are common in outpatient practice and are typically characterized by their historical characteristics. Cluster headaches tend to affect younger men. They are characterized by constant unilateral periorbital pain, lacrimation, and a blocked nostril. They tend to occur daily, often at night, for weeks or months. Migraines tend to be periodic and associated with nausea and vomiting. They are also unilateral, but typically throbbing. Classic migraines are preceded by a prodrome, usually visual. However, common migraines do not have the antecedent neurological symptoms. Migraines do not have the regular periodicity of a cluster. Tension headaches tend to be pressure-like, often times radiating from the neck over the top of the head, may come on with stress, and may last for days to weeks. Tumor-induced headaches, from increased intracranial pressure, tend to be progressive. They are characterized by no specific features. Nocturnal waking may be typical, but not diagnostic. Projectile vomiting may be present in the late stages. Sinus headaches are usually frontal or localized behind the eyes. Stooping, blowing the nose, and jarring the head may exacerbate the symptoms. (**Ref. 1,** p. 67)

20. **(B)** The clinical syndrome of arthritis, oral ulcerations, balanitis, and a rash consistent with keratoderma blenorrhagica is consistent with Reiter's syndrome. Of the disorders listed, the organism *Chlamydia trachomatis* is most closely associated with the development of Reiter's syndrome. Gonococcal arthritis is more of an inflammatory arthritis and the rash typically consists of isolated purplish vesicles with red bases. Psoriasis can have an arthritis similar to that of Reiter's syndrome. It is typically associated with the typical rash of psoriasis and pitting of the fingernails. Beta-hemolytic streptococcus is associated with rheumatic fever. Syphilis is more typically associated with ulcerations and rashes and less likely to have arthritis or tenosynovitis. (**Ref. 1,** p. 67)

21. (C) A number of drugs can interfere with the metabolism of warfarin. Therefore, any time a medication is added to a regimen containing warfarin, the potential impact on the prothrombin time should be considered. Antibiotics such as trimethoprim/sulfamethoxazole can have an impact on intestinal flora and, therefore, an indirect effect on the absorption of vitamin K. This frequently will lead to an increase in the warfarin levels and, therefore, the prothrombin time. Smoking has very little impact on the likelihood of prothrombin times changing. Cholestyramine can decrease the absorption of warfarin leading to a subtherapeutic prothrombin time. Similarly, a change in diet with additional green, leafy vegetables can increase the amount of vitamin K consumed and partially counteract the effect of warfarin. (**Ref. 1,** p. 812)

22. (C) The important aspects of this case are the positive straight leg raising test and the absent ankle jerk. Paraspinus muscle spasm is a non-specific finding which can be found in almost any injury to the back. Straight leg raising is most consistent with L-5 and S-1 radiculopathies. The absence of the ankle jerk suggests S-1 radiculopathy. L-4 nerve root irritation would have the greatest effect on the knee jerk. L-3 is a complex problem which may effect the knee jerk. Compression fractures have little or no impact on nerve roots unless there is impingement on the nerve root adjacent. L-5 lesions rarely cause a problem with lower extremity reflexes. (**Ref. 1,** pp. 73–74)

23. (D) Often a patient's family or friends do not wish to hear anything about a patient's suicidal thoughts. The opportunity to verbalize these feelings may be therapeutic. The remaining statements are myths that are not substantiated by empirical data. (**Ref. 10,** pp. 803–811)

24. (A) Her symptoms are consistent with criteria for major depressive disorder. There is not sufficient information to add "with melancholic features" which generally descibes a more severe depression. Dysthymic disorder is a less severe depression that has been going on for at least two years. There is no history of a manic episode to warrant a bipolar diagnosis although it is not impossible that she could have one in the future. Cyclothymic disorder again refers to moods swings of less severity and more chronicity. (**Ref. 16,** pp. 317–391)

25. (B) Efficacy is probably the least important factor because all antidepressants on the market are equally effective. Anticholinergic side effects may preclude a drug's use in the elderly. Drug-drug interactions may affect not just the choice of drugs but also the dose. Half-life affects dosing and the length of time the drug will remain in the body if another antidepressant is needed. Finally, cost is always a consideration, especially in this age of managed care. (**Ref. 11,** pp. 209–264)

26. (E) Actually, clomipramine is not solely an SSRI, but has strong serotonin properties. Its usual daily dose is 100 to 250 mgs. At the time of press, its approved indication is for obsessive compulsive disorder as is fluvoxamine. The remaining dose ranges are correct. (**Ref. 11,** p. 243)

27. (C) Selective Serotonin Reuptake Inhibitors (SSRI's) may cause decreased sexual desire and anorgasmia. Because decreased sexual drive may be a symptom of depression, its persistence after treatment is initiated may not be noticed by the physician unless the patient complains or is questioned directly. For some individuals, the sexual dysfunction side effects may be severe enough to warrant switching to another family of antidepressant. (**Ref. 21,** p. 171)

28. (A) The SSRI's are equally effective but are considerably more expensive than their predecessors. Their different side effect profiles have made them quite popular. They have considerably less anticholinergic side effects (dry mouth, constipation), and fewer cardiotoxic effects (which make them safer to prescribe in suicidal patients). Approximately 70% of people taking them report a stimulating effect, while the remainder report a sedating effect. (**Ref. 11,** pp. 280–281)

29. (E) The presenting symptoms and findings are common adverse effects associated with cocaine use. Cerebrovascular, epileptic, and cardiac effects are major complications of cocaine use. Death in cocaine users is often the result of seizures, cerebrovascular diseases, respiratory depression, and myocardial infarction that occur with high doses. (**Ref. 10,** pp. 426–427)

30. (B) The American Medical Association, the Accreditation Council for Continuing Medical Education, the American College of Physicians, and the Pharmaceutical Manufacturers Association all agree that it is unethical for physicians to accept direct payments to attend a meeting. It would be better for a company to support a conference so that a lower registration cost would permit more physicians to attend. (**Ref. 18,** pp. 301–305)

31. (C) The specifier with seasonal pattern can be added to several depressive diagnoses. In most cases the depression begins in the fall or winter and remits by spring. Individuals with a winter seasonal pattern are more often younger, female, and living in higher latitudes. (**Ref. 16,** p. 389)

32. (E) All the standard antidepressant medication therapies are reported to be effective in treating this condition. Phototherapy using bright lights has been reported to be effective, but remains experimental for now. However, since light boxes are not governed by the FDA, patients may purchase them without a prescription. Electroconvulsive therapy or ECT is generally reserved for depressions that have not responded to other treatments and is an effective mode of treatment. Anticonvulsants have not been demonstrated to be effective in unipolar depression. (**Ref. 11,** pp. 319–322)

33. (B) Duration of exposure is important and is inversely proportional to the intensity. A half-hour exposure to 10,000 lux may be equivalent to a two-hour exposure to 2,500 lux. (**Ref. 11,** p. 320)

34. (D) This case presents with several issues. Daytime urinary incontinence in children after 4 years of age and nighttime incontinence after 6 years of age is defined as enuresis. Despite this definition, it is not unusual for nighttime enuresis to persist to 7 to 8 years of age. However, once a child has been continent for over three months, return of enuresis is defined as secondary enuresis and is often associated with an acute psychosocial stressor, such as the birth of a baby, a family death, or changes in the family dynamics. Appropriate therapy for enuresis includes positive reinforcement, minimizing the impact on the child's self-esteem, and recognition that most enuresis (especially secondary enursesis) resolves spontaneously. The use of medications is associated with side effects and has not been shown to improve long-term results. **(Ref. 6,** pp. 107–108)

35. (E) Routine administration of available immunizations has resulted in marked decreases in morbidity and mortality for a variety of infectious diseases. Despite few absolute contraindications, delay of immunizations is a significant problem. Providing appropriate immunizations when children present is an important role in pediatric preventive health initiatives. The recommended immunization schedule for children not immunized in the first year of life has been developed by the Committee on Infectious Diseases of the American Academy of Pediatrics. There is no contraindication to administering the DTP, Hib vaccine, hepatovax, MMR, and polio vaccines at the initial setting. (Recent concerns about transmission of the live vaccine administered in the OPV may result in the recommendation for the first two polio vaccines to be provided as the inactivated form, IPV.) In addition, if the child is at high risk for exposure to tuberculosis, a tuberculin skin test should also be applied. **(Ref. 6,** p. 31)

36. (B) Trisomy 21 (Down's syndrome) is the most common chromosomal abnormality seen in live births. Up to half of children with trisomy 21 have congenital heart disease. Abnormalities in growth are nearly universal and have resulted in the development of growth charts specific to children with Down's syndrome. The abnormalities in growth are apparent at an early age, are not associated with delays in bone age, and do not appear to be secondary to abnormalities of growth hormone. Both hypothyroidism and congenital heart disease can exacerbate the short stature seen in these children. (**Ref. 6,** pp. 297–299, 1699–1700)

37. (A) Children with trisomy 21 are at risk for increased difficulties involving a variety of medical problems. The incidence of hearing loss approaches 50%. Children with trisomy 21 are at increased risk of developing leukemia, diabetes, hypothyroidism, and cataracts. There is no evidence that atherosclerotic disease appears more rapidly nor that they have an increased risk of caries, but the pathologic features of Alzheimer's disease often appear in these patients as early as the fourth decade. (**Ref. 6,** pp. 297–299)

38. (E) Endocardial cushion defects are due to arrested development of the endocardial cushions leading to failure of the embryological development of distinct tricuspid and mitral valve rings and development of a ventricular septal defect. While children with trisomy 21 often have a more favorable anatomy for correction, persistence of abnormal valves is common. Indications for prophylaxis include children with congenital heart disease and appropriate antibiotics must be prescribed prior to dental therapy. (**Ref. 6,** pp. 1470, 1526)

5

Other Encounters

DIRECTIONS (Questions 1–29): Each of the numbered items or incomplete statements in this chapter is followed by answers or completions of the statement. Select the **ONE** lettered answer or completion that is **BEST** in each case.

1. An 11-year-old was just thrown over the handlebars of his bicycle and sustained a few abrasions as well as complete evulsion of his right maxillary incisor tooth. The appropriate advice to this family is

   A. no actions are necessary as this is a primary tooth and will be replaced with natural eruption of the permanent tooth

   B. find the tooth and after rinsing it in water bring it (and the child) to your office immediately

   C. find the tooth, rinse it in water, pack the gum with wet towels, and take the child to the dentist

   D. find the tooth, rinse it off, and place it in milk to preserve the periodontal ligaments; arrange to see the dentist within the next 24 hours

   E. find the tooth, rinse it in water, replace it carefully in the socket; take the child to the dentist immediately

2. The mother of a 6-year-old known diabetic calls for advice. He vomited once yesterday and now has diarrhea, with watery stools occurring every two to three hours. He had decrease in appetite but feels he'll eat well this morning. His blood glucose measurements, measured prior to every meal, have ranged from 80 mg/dL before supper last evening to 320 mg/dL this morning. Urine ketones have been present in trace amounts since last evening. His normal insulin doses include:

   4 U regular insulin and 10 U NPH before breakfast

   2 U regular and 5 U NPH before dinner

   The appropriate intervention for the treatment of this child's hyperglycemia is

   A. decrease his intake of food and administer the usual insulin dose before breakfast; increase the monitoring of blood glucose levels

   B. provide the usual morning insulin and breakfast, increasing the NPH provided with dinner; increase the monitoring of blood glucose levels

   C. increase this morning's NPH and provide the usual breakfast

   D. increase this morning's regular insulin, provide the usual breakfast, and increase monitoring

   E. hold this morning's NPH, providing the usual breakfast

3. While on call, you receive a phone call from the mother of a 5-month-old who has had "the flu" for the last 24 hours. She vomited several times yesterday and has developed diarrhea early this morning. By history, the child has had stools (without blood or mucus) every two to three hours. She appears thirsty. She is sleeping more than usual but will awaken and is restless when awake. There are tears present during crying but her mucous membranes are slightly dry. She has had several wet diapers since last evening. Her soft spot does not appear sunken to Mom. She is afebrile. After discussing the signs and symptoms, appropriate advice for the mother may include all of the following **EXCEPT**

A. take the child to the ER immediately for treatment of dehydration

B. provide frequent feedings of diluted cola, making sure she takes at least 2 ounces every hour

C. stop all feeding until the stooling diminishes, then begin clear liquids

D. initiate oral rehydration using Pedialyte, watching for signs of persistent dehydration

E. initiate regular feedings, encouraging larger quantities of water

4. The mother of a 2-year-old calls after office hours. She has just been notified that her child was exposed to another child with meningitis at daycare. The mother is extremely concerned that her child may contract the disease. The most appropriate next step is to

A. call the pharmacy with a prescription for rifampin prophylaxis

B. reassure the mother that most forms of meningitis are viral and there's nothing to do but watch for fever and lethargy

C. discover the name of the hospital or doctor caring for the child with meningitis to obtain more information

D. call the pharmacy with a prescription for a course of penicillin to prevent development of meningitis

E. arrange for the mother to bring her child to the office in the morning for a physical examination and evaluation

5. A 4-year-old fell backwards from a height of approximately two feet, landing on his buttocks but striking the back of his head as well. His mother calls you for advice on what to do next. The information which would suggest the need for immediate evaluation includes

   A. he cried immediately and then vomited once shortly after being calmed

   B. there is a half-dollar-sized area of swelling over the occiput of his head

   C. he appeared stunned after the fall, but was responsive to verbal stimulation

   D. there is a small cut over the back of his head that stopped bleeding with minimal pressure

   E. he was unarousable for several minutes and now seems somewhat lethargic

Case Cluster (Questions 6–7):

6. Your receptionist gives you a message from a 29-year-old female who has called your office complaining of vaginal bleeding. You return the call in a timely manner. She explains she has had heavy vaginal bleeding for the last three days after missing her period one week ago. She states she is passing quarter-sized clots but no tissue. She denies fever but feels somewhat lightheaded. She denies sexual activity and uses no contraception. You offer to

   A. give her an appointment in your office as soon as possible that day

   B. make her an appointment with a gynecologist sometime in the next few days

C. call in a prescription for 0.625 mg of estrogen with 10 mg of progesterone a day for ten days

D. see her if the problem recurs next month because you tell her the heavy bleeding is the result of her missing her regularly scheduled menstrual cycle

E. tell her to maintain bedrest and call for an appointment for the next day if the bleeding continues

7. She elects to see you the following morning. Initial vital signs include a blood pressure of 112/68 and pulse 80 standing, 110/66 and pulse 72 sitting, respirations 18/min and temperature of 98°. Her examination is benign except pelvic exam which reveals a vaginal vault with blood and small clots and no tissue. Cervical os slightly open with no tissue but with a small amount of blood. Uterus is not enlarged or tender. Left adnexa is slightly enlarged but not tender and no discrete mass is appreciated. Right adnexa is normal. There is no evidence of trauma or infection from visual or manual inspection. She requests that you order as few tests as possible because she has no health insurance. You decide the test that will best help you in management of her problems is

A. CBC

B. quantitative βHCG

C. cervical cultures for gonorrhea and chlamydia

D. endometrial aspiration biopsy

E. pelvic ultrasound

Case Cluster (Questions 8–11):

8. Your receptionist gives you a message from a 50-year-old female who has been your patient for the last ten years. She is requesting medicine for anxiety. You call her back in a timely manner. She explains she is having problems at work that are causing her anxiety. She cannot take time off to come in because she is afraid of losing her job. Although she has not been in to the health center for the last year, her chart documents no problems with substance abuse, domestic violence, depression, or anxiety. Although you sympathize with her situation, you are worried about prescribing medications without evaluating her in the office. The soonest evening appointment (that way she won't miss any work) that you can offer her is in two weeks. She says that would be fine and work out well for her. Although all of the following can contribute to anxiety, which item is *essential* to assess before hanging up?

   A. Substance abuse

   B. Domestic violence

   C. Suicide potential

   D. Menopause status

   E. Insomnia

9. You see the patient in two weeks. Although she claims to be less anxious because her work situation has improved, she says she is worried about her menstrual problems. After having no menstrual bleeding for one year, she has had two weeks of light intermittent spotting. She is not sexually active although living with her spouse. Important in your initial evaluation are all of the following **EXCEPT**

   A. pelvic examination

   B. assay for LH and FSH

C. endometrial aspiration

D. ultrasound of endometrial stripe

E. βHCG

10. After you have finished conducting a thorough assessment of her menstrual irregularity over the next few weeks, it is benign. You decide to discuss hormone replacement therapy. A family history of which of the following conditions would make hormone replacement therapy (HRTx) even more advisable in this particular patient?

   A. Diabetes and coronary artery disease

   B. Osteoporosis and coronary artery disease

   C. Diabetes and osteoporosis

   D. Depression and osteoporosis

   E. Osteoporosis and hypertension

11. Before prescribing hormones, you tell your patient you would like her to get which of the following tests?

   A. Mammogram

   B. CBC

   C. Fasting lipid panel

   D. FSH and LH assay

   E. TSH

Case Clusters (Questions 12–15):

12. The nursing home calls you about evaluation and management of one of your elderly female patients who resides there. Ms. X is 84 years old. She is not demented but has been residing at the nursing home for the last month for rehabilitation after hip replacement. Other than Coumadin, she is on no medication. She has been progressing well with her rehabilitation and now is able to walk with the assistance of a walker. She has no chronic diseases such as hypertension, diabetes, or coronary artery disease, and has never had a stroke. The nurse at the nursing home tells you she has been "losing her urine more frequently" for the last four days. Differential diagnosis includes all of the following **EXCEPT**

    A. urge incontinence

    B. stress incontinence

    C. fecal impaction

    D. estrogen deficiency

    E. urinary tract infection

13. Prior to visiting the patient, it would be appropriate to order all of the following lab tests **EXCEPT**

    A. urinalysis

    B. urine culture

    C. CBC

    D. FSH, LH

    E. fasting blood sugar

14. After your examination of the patient and a review of her lab tests you decide the patient's difficulty with ambulation prevents her from using the toilet appropriately. The most important first step would be to offer which of the following interventions or medications to improve this patient's continence?

    A. Oxybutynin

    B. Foley catheter at night

    C. Estrogen therapy

    D. Bladder training

    E. Imipramine

15. Other interventions or medications might include all of the following **EXCEPT**

    A. regulation of bowel elimination

    B. commode at the bedside

    C. indwelling urinary catheter

    D. estrogen therapy

    E. imipramine

16. One of your well-informed patients questions you about a magazine article she read that stated that hormone replacement therapy has been strongly recommended as a clinical prevention strategy for all postmenopausal women by many professional health care organizations. You inform her that contraindications include all of the following **EXCEPT**

   A.   breast cancer

   B.   cancer of the endometrium

   C.   coronary artery disease

   D.   thromboembolic disease

   E.   undiagnosed vaginal bleeding

Case Cluster (Quesions 17–18):

17. A colleague consults with you regarding a patient of his who is a 42-year-old married white woman with newly diagnosed breast cancer and palpable axillary lymph nodes. He asks you how often histologic evaluation fails to reveal malignancy. You reply that this occurs in approximately

   A.   5% of cases

   B.   15% of cases

   C.   25% of cases

   D.   35% of cases

   E.   none of the above

18. He asks you about the ten-year local control rate for a breast carcinoma less than 5 cm in diameter treated by excisional biopsy and primary radiotherapy. You reply that the control rate is approximately

   A. 90%–95%

   B. 80%–85%

   C. 70%–75%

   D. 60%–65%

   E. < 50%

19. A 62-year-old woman stops you after a public lecture on osteoporosis. She asks you about risk factors. All of the following factors increase the risk of symptomatic osteoporosis in women **EXCEPT**

   A. low initial bone density

   B. premature menopause

   C. a diet containing 1000–1500 mg/day of elemental calcium

   D. smoking and heavy alcohol use

   E. long-term intake of phenytoin or glucocorticoids

20. Which of the following patients is **LEAST** likely to have sudden death?

    A. A 55-year-old man with severe three-vessel coronary artery disease

    B. A 35-year-old man with a cardial myopathy and an injection fraction of 30%

    C. A 65-year-old man with frequent PVC's and good left ventricle function by dobutamine stress ECHO

    D. A 55-year-old cigarette smoker with hypercholesterolemia, hypertension, diabetes mellitus, and EKG evidence of LVH

    E. A 62-year-old woman one year after a subendocardial myocardial infarction

21. An 82-year-old white female, nursing home resident, develops mental status changes. Her serum sodium is low at 120 mg/dl. Urine osmolarity is high at 300. Which of the medications on her medications list is most likely responsible?

    A. Trimethoprim

    B. Enalapril

    C. Digoxin

    D. Chlorpropamide

    E. Lithium carbonate

22. Which of the following patients does **NOT** require prophylaxis when seeing the dentist for a tooth cleaning?

    A. A 68-year-old man with a transvenous cardiac pacemaker

    B. A 42-year-old woman with a prosthetic aortic valve

C. A 28-year-old black man with a patent ventricular septal defect

D. A 78-year-old woman with mitral insufficiency

E. A 50-year-old woman with previous valvular endocarditis

23. You are seeing an 82-year-old white woman as a new patient in your clinic. All of the following findings are consistent with normal aging, **EXCEPT**

A. significant reduction in glomerular filtration rate (GFR)

B. decreased colonic motility with constipation

C. early morning awakening and insomnia

D. elevation of the fasting blood glucose to 140 to 160 mg %

E. changes in the "set point" for vasopressin release so SIADH is more likely

24. A 77-year-old white woman is evaluated in the nursing home for shaking spells. She is noted to have a mild resting tremor which worsens on reaching for a cup of water or pointing her finger. The likely diagnosis is

A. peripheral myopathy

B. Parkinson's disease

C. essential familial tremor

D. basal ganglia infarcts

E. Wilson's disease

25. A 73-year-old black woman is brought into the office by her anxious daughter. She has been refusing medications, wandering out of the house, and forgetting to eat. She is being treated for hypertension and congestive heart failure. All of the following statements are true **EXCEPT**

    A. multiinfarct dementia is frequently difficult to distinguish from Alzheimer's disease

    B. severe depression may be responsible

    C. evaluation should include a CBC, metabolic screen (SMA 12–20), serum TSH, B 12, VDRL, and CT or MRI brain scan

    D. a toxicologic drug screen may be useful

    E. the likelihood of finding a reversible cause is approximately 30%

Case Cluster (Questions 26–27):

26. You are making your regular morning visit to the nursing home where you consult. The nursing staff informs you that your 72-year-old patient becomes increasingly confused after supper each day. You examine the patient and she calmly tells you she feels fine. She is oriented to person, place, and time. The term that best describes this situation is

    A. catastrophic reaction

    B. sundowner syndrome

    C. dementia of the Alzheimer's type

    D. vascular dementia

    E. major depressive disorder

27. Your next action should be

    A. referral to a psychiatrist

    B. referral to a neurologist

    C. a comprehensive laboratory workup

    D. simply have staff observe for any further deterioration

    E. reassure the family that this is a normal part of aging

Case Cluster (Questions 28–29):

28. A 78-year-old nursing home resident has been thinking about what would happen to her if a debilitating illness struck. Her cardiac condition has been stable, her diabetes is under control, and it has been four years since her right foot has been amputated. She has mentioned to other residents of the nursing home that she "would never wish to be attached to a machine." The following are characteristics of a trustworthy oral advanced directive **EXCEPT**

    A. the preferences of the patient are informed

    B. the directive reviews specific treatments and clinical situations

    C. the patient makes a choice about future health care

    D. the patient expresses a desire to have control over future health care decisions

    E. the directive is changed on a regular basis

29. The most comprehensive and flexible advanced directive is

    A. oral statement to family

    B. oral statement to friends

    C. oral statement to personal physician

    D. durable power of attorney for health care

    E. living will

Other Encounters

Answers and Discussion

1. **(E)** Approximately 10% of all children will sustain significant dental trauma during childhood. If an avulsed tooth is replanted within 30 minutes of the injury, over 90% of teeth are viable. If the tooth is not replaced within two hours, over 95% of those teeth will be lost. Rinsing the tooth in water and replacing it in the socket immediately is the correct choice. Immediate examination by the dentist should also be performed. If the family members are uncomfortable replacing the tooth, transporting it in milk will maintain the viability of the periodontal ligament. The viability of this ligament is vital to successful replantation of the tooth. (**Ref. 5,** pp. 1047–1048)

2. **(D)** Close monitoring of blood glucose and attention to detail is crucial in the management of diabetes during an intercurrent illness. The presence of urinary ketones, even in the face of normal blood glucose levels, suggests inadequate insulin supplementation and should result in an increased dose of regular insulin. Regular insulin has an onset of 30 minutes, peak action at two to three hours, and four to six hour duration of action. Human NPH has a slower onset (2 to 3 hours) with a peak action at six to ten hours. When otherwise healthy, a repeatedly elevated morning blood glucose should result in an increase in the p.m. NPH dose. However, while ill and with ketones in the urine, the appropriate action is to increase the dose of regular insulin, increase fluids, and evaluate the response with increased monitoring. (**Ref. 6,** pp. 1811–1813)

3. **(C)** Gastroenteritis is a leading cause of dehydration. Assessing the degree of dehydration by history requires careful attention to detail, looking for evidence of decreased intravascular volume including markedly decreased urination, decreased tearing, and evidence of altered mental status. This child's signs and symptoms are consistent with mild to moderate dehydration and would allow the use of oral rehydration. The inability to retain any fluids is an indication for evaluation and the possible need for IV rehydration. As this child's emesis has resolved, the choice of rehydrating solution needs to be addressed. Dehydration is accompanied by increased losses of sodium and potassium. Therefore, rehydration should be performed using solutions with reasonable concentrations of these ions. Water has little of either ion and diluted cola is low in both sodium and potassium. While stopping feedings in the face of diarrhea is a common practice, doing so in this child who already has signs and symptoms of dehydration is counterproductive. (**Ref. 5,** pp. 209–213)

4. **(C)** Prophylaxis with rifampin for meningitis exposure is recommended only for contacts exposed to meningitis caused by *Neisseria meningitidis* and hemophilus influenza, type B. Viral meningitis is more common than bacterial and is not responsive to prophylactic therapy. Determining the etiology of the meningitis is important prior to instituting therapy. Discussing the signs and symptoms to watch for is important but examination is not necessary unless symptomatology exists. (**Ref. 5,** p. 713)

5. **(E)** Head injury is a frequent occurrence in the pediatric population. Fortunately, the majority of head injuries are mild. Indications for evaluation include a large scalp laceration, an obvious deformity of the skull, loss of consciousness, or persistent neurological abnormality. It is common for children to vomit after even mild head injury. Persistent vomiting requires further evaluation. Children who experience a loss of consciousness (a concussion) should be evaluated and observed until there is a full recovery of consciousness. (**Ref. 6,** pp. 1932–1934)

6. **(A)** Although the patient denies sexual activity, one must always maintain a healthy suspicion in cases of late and heavy menstrual flow. Ectopic pregnancy or spontaneous abortion can present in this manner. Rather than waiting to see if the bleeding occurs with the next cycle or referring her to a gynecologist in a few days, it is prudent to see the patient as soon as possible and rule out pregnancy with a β-HCG. Although conjugated estrogens and progesterone can be used to regulate menstrual flow, you must first see the patient and rule out ectopic pregnancy or miscarriage. (**Ref. 9,** p. 536)

7. **(B)** Dysfuntional uterine bleeding is a diagnosis of exclusion. You must first and foremost rule out pregnancy and pregnancy-related problems (ectopic pregnancy or spontaneous abortion) with a β-HCG. Polycystic ovarian syndrome, cancers of cervix and endometrium, blood dyscrasias, thyroid problems, and a variety of medications can also cause abnormal uterine bleeding. These diagnoses can be pursued once the β-HCG is found to be negative. (**Ref. 9,** p. 536)

8. **(C)** Although the patient seems content to wait two weeks for an evening appointment, don't forget to assess her suicide potential before hanging up. Suicidal patients often talk to their physicians before attempting or succeeding at suicide. They may be hesitant or afraid to discuss the depth of their depression and suicide ideation. It is essential that you ask anxious or depressed patients whether they have thought about suicide. Substance abuse, domestic violence, and menopause can all be contributing factors to anxiety. However, you can assess these later when you see the patient. (**Ref. 20,** p. 161)

9. **(B)** As assay for LH and/or FSH does not help you determine the cause of your patient's vaginal bleeding. A pelvic examination is necessary to look for abnormalities such as lacerations, infections, or cancers which can lead to bleeding. Endometrial cancer must be excluded in any woman of perimenopausal age who has endome-

trial bleeding after a six-month cessation of menstrual flow. An ultrasound of the endometrial stripe or endometrial aspiration can be helpful in determining the presence of endometrial cancer. Finally, although the patient denies sexual activity, it is important to exclude pregnancy. (**Ref. 9,** p. 593)

10. **(B)** Hormone replacement therapy is effective in both decreasing the progression of osteoporosis if started at menopause and also preventing atherosclerosis. Protection against both coronary artery disease and cerebrovascular accidents is a major benefit of estrogen replacement. A family history of atherosclerotic disease or osteoporosis makes hormone replacement therapy even more advisable. (**Ref. 9,** pp. 595–611)

11. **(A)** Since there is still considerable controversy surrounding the link between breast cancer and estrogen replacement, breast cancer must be ruled out prior to initiating therapy. In addition, for women over 50 years of age, annual mammography is indicated as a clinical prevention strategy. (**Ref. 9,** pp. 612–616)

12. **(A)** Incontinence in the elderly can result from different mechanisms or pathologies. Urge incontinence is common in patients with dementia or after a stroke. It results from detrusor instability and an inability by the patient to suppress the detrusor muscle contraction when the bladder is full. Your patient is not demented and has not had a stroke as far as you know. Overflow incontinence refers to the opposite problem of decreased detrusor activity which occurs as a result of diabetic neuropathy or prostatic hypertrophy. The bladder becomes overdistended and overflows. Functional incontinence, mentioned later in the question series, results from mobility impairment or from medications such as diuretics. Patients who have functional incontinence have normal voiding mechanisms. Stress incontinence refers to urinary sphincter insufficiency. Patients lose their urine involuntarily when they cough or laugh. It is common in women who have sustained perineal trauma during childbirth or who are postmenopausal. Estrogen deficiency in the postmenopausal woman can amplify stress incontinence. Fecal impaction causes undue stress on the bladder; it is

common in elderly nursing home residents especially post-operatively. Urinary tract infection is a common cause of urinary incontinence. (**Ref. 20,** pp. 79–84)

13. (**D**) Although the postmenopausal state can be detected with FSH and LH assays, it is unnecessary to order in elderly nonmenstruating females. Hyperglycemia with glycosuria or diabetes can lead to incontinence. Urinary tract infections can be detected with a urinalysis or urine culture. An elevated white blood count can help detect occult infection of any sort which might lead to incontinence by affecting mental status or mobility. (**Ref. 20,** pp. 79–84)

14. (**D**) From the history, one can assume that the patient's incontinence stems from somewhat impaired immobility after her operation and probably estrogen deficiency with resulting stress incontinence. The first steps in treating this type of incontinence consist of bladder retraining, after ruling out reversible causes like fecal impaction, medications, or urinary tract infections. Foley catheters have no place in initial management unless skin ulceration is present. (**Ref. 20,** pp. 79–84)

15. (**C**) Indwelling Foley catheters have no place in managing incontinence unless skin maceration or ulceration is present. Imipramine can be helpful in patients with sphincter insufficiency (stress incontinence). Estrogen can decrease vaginal atrophy and also improve sphincter tone, thereby improving continence. Regulation of bowel elimination and providing easier access to the toilet with a commode can also improve continence. (**Ref. 20,** pp. 79–84)

16. (**C**) In well controlled hypertension, hormone replacement therapy can be prescribed. In fact, since hormone replacement therapy has been shown to decrease coronary artery disease, the combination of estrogen and antihypertensive medications along with aspirin have added benefit in preventing coronary artery disease. (**Ref. 21,** p. 1306)

17. **(C)** Physical examination yields a false-positive (enlarged nodes that are histologically negative) rate of approximately 25% in breast cancer patients with palpable axillary nodes. Similarly, in the absence of adenopathy on physical exam, pathologic examination reveals metastatic tumor in approximately 30% of cases (false-negative). The presence of histologically involved lymph nodes is the most important powerful predictor of future recurrence. (**Ref. 20,** pp. 1326–1328)

18. **(A)** Multiple retrospective and prospective studies have shown excellent control of the primary tumor in stage I (< 2 cm) and stage II (2–5 cm) breast cancer. Long-term survival is equivalent to that obtained by modified radical mastectomy. (**Ref. 20,** pp. 1326–1328)

19. **(C)** It is recommended that all premenopausal and post-menopausal women consume 1000–1500 mg/day of elemental calcium; however, the average calcium intake of postmenopausal American women is only 550 mg/day. The low initial bone density of white and Asian women increases their risk of osteoporosis as compared with black women. The estrogen deficiency of premature menopause results in earlier onset of osteoporosis. Smoking, heavy alcohol intake, and chronic phenytoin and glucocorticoid therapy are other important risk factors. Prophylactic or preventive therapy with estrogen will have the greatest benefit/toxicity ratio in high-risk individuals. (**Ref. 9,** p. 599)

20. **(C)** Sudden cardiac death has been associated with previous myocardial infarction; three-vessel or left main equivalent coronary artery disease; impaired left ventricular function, especially when it is associated with cardiomyopathy; and the usual cardiac risk factors such as smoking, hyperlipidemia, hypertension, and diabetes. The presence of frequent premature ventricular contractions in the presence of good left ventricular function is not considered to be a risk factor. (**Ref. 1,** pp. 192–195)

21. **(D)** The pattern of the low serum sodium and the high urine osmolarity indicates that this person has the syndrome of inappro-

priate antidiuretic hormone secretion (SIADH). Hypoglycemic drugs such as tolbutamide and chlorpropamide are capable of inducing a SIADH-like syndrome. Lithium carbonate tends to effect tubular handling of sodium. Drugs such as trimethoprim, enalapril, or digoxin have no significant impact on sodium metabolism. (**Ref. 1,** pp. 1928–1929)

22. **(A)** Prosthetic valve, patent ventricular septal defect, and mitral valve leisons, and patients with a previous history of endocarditis are all at relatively high risk for developing bacterial endocarditis. In the setting of high-risk procedures, such as dental work, these patients should receive prophylaxis. Transvenous pacemakers, however, are very low risk for developing endocarditis and no prophylaxis is necessary. (**Ref. 1,** pp. 525–526)

23. **(D)** There are a number of changes that are consistent with normal aging. Reduction in glomerular filtration rate, decreased colonic motility, early awakening and insomnia, and changes in osmotic regulation can all be relatively normal findings. These changes should be considered when selecting medications for older patients so as to avoid exacerbating the problem, or causing inappropriate accumulation of medication. Elevation of the fasting blood glucose to greater than 140 is abnormal and a diagnosis of diabetes mellitus should be considered in the geriatric patient as well as the younger patient. (**Ref. 1,** p. 31)

24. **(C)** The tremor described is known as an action tremor. Parkinson's disease and Wilson's disease typically have a resting tremor. Basal ganglia infarcts can have a rolling motion that is not consistent with an action tremor as described here. The tremor described is most typically seen in benign essential familial tremor. (**Ref. 1,** p. 123)

25. **(A)** Multiinfarct dementia from cerebral vascular disease can cause about 20% of progressive dementias. It is usually easily differentiated from Alzheimer's disease, because of its stuttering progression, focal motor symptoms, and signs in the presence of

multiple infarctions on a CT or MRI brain scan. Alzheimer's, which causes 50% to 60% of dementias, can be diagnosed with 90% accuracy using history, physical examination, and the laboratory tests listed. A careful drug history, occasionally supplemented by toxicologic drug screen, will rule out chronic drug intoxication. Careful history and examination are needed to rule out depression, which may mimic dementia or complicate it and exacerbate it. Only approximately 30% of dementias have a reversible cause; 10% have treatable neurologic or systemic illness, 10% are pseudo dementias, such as depression, and 10% may have a modifiable contributing cause which can be improved. (**Ref. 1,** p. 145)

26. **(B)** The waxing and waning of mental status is not uncommon when there is an organic etiology. Confusion, ataxia, drowsiness, and accidental falls can occur in elderly patients who are oversedated and in demented patients in the evening when there is reduced external stimuli, including light and other people (such as staff). (**Ref. 10,** p. 353)

27. **(C)** Whenever a patient is suspected of having dementia, a comprehensive laboratory workup must be initiated to eliminate possible reversible causes of the dementia. It will also provide the patient and family with a more definitive diagnosis. The exam should include a physical examination, vitals, formal mental status examination, medication review, drug levels, blood and urine screens for alcohol, drugs, and heavy metals, physiologic workup, chest x-ray, EKG, neurological workup, and neuropsychological testing. (**Ref. 10,** pp. 353–357)

28. **(E)** An oral advanced directive is considered more trustworthy if the "directive is repeated over time, in different situations, to various individuals." It is this consistency that makes it more probable that the decision is considered carefully and based on preferences deeply held. Such patients are unlikely to change their minds about these directives. (**Ref. 18,** pp. 95–99)

29. (D) The durable power of attorney is more flexible and comprehensive because it applies to all situations in which a person is incapable of making decisions, not just at the end of life. Together with a statement indicating preferences about life-sustaining treatments, this is the preferred method of advanced directive. Several states have specifically passed legislation authorizing this. In contrast, living wills have specific limitations and oral directives have been rejected by courts in some states. (**Ref. 18,** pp. 97–102)

References

1. Isselbacher, et al. eds. *Harrison's Principles of Internal Medicine.* ed. 13. New York: McGraw Hill, 1994.

2. Cecil, et al. eds. *Cecil Textbook of Medicine.* ed. 20. Philadelphia, PA: WB Saunders Co, 1996.

3. Tierney LM, et al., *Current Medical Diagnosis and Treatment.* ed. 35. Stamford, CT: Appleton and Lange, 1996.

4. Goroll AH, et al. *Primary Care Medicine: Office evaluation and management of the adult patient.* ed. 3. Philadelphia, PA: Lippincott, 1995.

5. Behrmen RE, Kliegman RN. *Nelson Essentials of Pediatrics.* ed. 2. Philadelphia, PA: Saunders, 1994.

6. Rudolph AM, ed. *Rudolph's Pediatrics.* ed. 20. Stamford, CT: Appleton & Lange, 1996.

7. Green M, Haggerty RT, eds. *Ambulatory Pediatrics IV.* Philadelphia, PA: Saunders, 1990.

8. Cunningham, et al. *William's Obstetrics.* ed. 19. Stamford, CT: Appleton & Lange, 1993.

9. Speroff L. *Clinical Gynecologic Endocrinology and Infertility.* ed. 5. Baltimore: Williams & Wilkins, 1994.

10. Kaplan H, Sadock B, Grebb, J. *Kaplan & Sadock's Synopsis of Psychiatry.* ed. 7. Baltimore: Williams & Wilkins, 1994.

11. Janicak, et al., *Principles & Practice of Psychopharmacotherapy.* Baltimore: Williams & Wilkins, 1993.

12. Rosen P, Barkin RM. *Emergency Medicine, Concepts and Clinical Practice.* St. Louis, MO: Mosby Year Book, 1992.

13. Strange GR, Ahrens W, Lelyveld S, Schafermeyer R, American College of Emergency Physicians. *Pediatric Emergency Medicine, A Comprehensive Study Guide.* New York: McGraw-Hill, 1996.

14. Schwartz S. *Principles of Surgery.* New York: McGraw-Hill, 1994.

15. Tintinalli JE, Ruiz E, Krome RL, American College of Emergency Physicians. *Emergency Medicine, A Comprehensive Study Guide.* New York: McGraw-Hill, 1996.